The Practice of Catheter Cryoablation
for Cardiac Arrhythmias

To my wife, Lillian, and my little daughter, Nam Nam, for bringing me a new page of life.

– NY

The Practice of Catheter Cryoablation for Cardiac Arrhythmias

EDITED BY

Ngai-Yin Chan, MBBS, FRCP, FACC, FHRS

Head, Cardiac Pacing Service and
Head, Cardiac Rehabilitation Service
Department of Medicine and Geriatrics
Princess Margaret Hospital
Hong Kong
China

WILEY Blackwell

Library of Congress Cataloging-in-Publication Data

The practice of catheter cryoablation for cardiac arrhythmias / edited by Ngai-Yin Chan.
       p. ; cm.
    Includes bibliographical references and index.
    ISBN 978-1-118-45183-0 (cloth : alk. paper) – ISBN 978-1-118-45179-3 – ISBN 978-1-118-45180-9 (Mobi) – ISBN 978-1-118-45181-6 (Pdf) – ISBN 978-1-118-45182-3 (ePub) – ISBN 978-1-118-75776-5 – ISBN 978-1-118-75777-2
    I. Chan, Ngai-Yin, editor of compilation.
    [DNLM: 1. Arrhythmias, Cardiac–surgery.   2. Catheter Ablation–methods. 3. Cryosurgery–methods. WG 330]
    RC685.A65
    616.1'28–dc23
                                           2013017939

A catalogue record for this book is available from the British Library.

Cover image: courtesy of the editor
Cover design by Rob Sawkins for Opta Design Ltd.

Set in 9/12 Photina MT by Toppan Best-set Premedia Limited
Printed and bound in Malaysia by Vivar Printing Sdn Bhd

1   2014

Contents

List of Contributors

Amin Al-Ahmad, MD
Division of Cardiovascular Medicine
Stanford University School of Medicine
Palo Alto, CA
USA

David J. Burkhardt, MD
Texas Cardiac Arrhythmia Institute
St. David's Medical Center
Austin, TX
USA

Ngai-Yin Chan, MBBS, FRCP, FACC, FHRS
Department of Medicine and Geriatrics
Princess Margaret Hospital
Hong Kong
China

Kathryn K. Collins, MD
University of Colorado and
Children's Hospital Colorado
Aurora, CO
USA

Luigi Di Biase, MD, PhD, FHRS
Texas Cardiac Arrhythmia Institute
St. David's Medical Center;
Department of Biomedical Engineering
University of Texas
Austin, TX
USA;
Department of Cardiology
University of Foggia
Foggia
Italy;
Albert Einstein College of Medicine
Montefiore Hospital
New York, NY
USA

Gregory K. Feld, MD
Clinical Cardiac Electrophysiology Program
Division of Cardiology
University of California, San Diego
San Diego, CA;
Sulpizio Family Cardiovascular Center
La Jolla, CA
USA

Jo Jo Hai, MBBS
Cardiology Division
Department of Medicine
Queen Mary Hospital
The University of Hong Kong
Hong Kong
China

Henry H. Hsia, MD
Division of Cardiovascular Medicine
Stanford University School of Medicine
Palo Alto, CA
USA

Marcin Kowalski, MD, FHRS
Department of Clinical Cardiac Electrophysiology
Staten Island University Hospital
Staten Island, NY
USA

Michael R. Lauer, MD
Permanente Medical Group
Cardiac Electrophysiology Laboratory
Kaiser-Permanente Medical Center
San Jose, CA
USA

Andrea Natale, MD, FACC, FHRS
Texas Cardiac Arrhythmia Institute
St. David's Medical Center;
Department of Biomedical Engineering
University of Texas
Austin, TX;
Division of Cardiovascular Medicine
Stanford University School of Medicine
Palo Alto, CA;
Sutter Pacific Medical Center
San Francisco, CA
USA

Pasquale Santangeli, MD
Texas Cardiac Arrhythmia Institute
St. David's Medical Center
Austin, TX
USA;
Department of Cardiology
University of Foggia
Foggia
Italy;
Division of Cardiovascular Medicine
Stanford University School of Medicine
Palo Alto, CA
USA

Navinder Sawhney, MD
Cardiac Electrophysiology Program
Division of Cardiology
University of California, San Diego
San Diego, CA;
Sulpizio Family Cardiovascular Center
La Jolla, CA
USA

Ruey J. Sung, MD
Division of Cardiovascular Medicine (Emeritus)
Stanford University School of Medicine
Stanford, CA
USA

Hung-Fat Tse, MD, PhD
Cardiology Division
Department of Medicine
Queen Mary Hospital
The University of Hong Kong
Hong Kong
China

George F. Van Hare, MD
Division of Pediatric Cardiology
Washington University School of Medicine and
St. Louis Children's Hospital
St. Louis, MO
USA

Jürgen Vogt, MD
Department of Cardiology
Heart and Diabetes Center North Rhine-Westphalia
Ruhr University Bochum
Bad Oeynhausen
Germany

Xue Yan
Department of Biomedical Engineering
Texas Cardiac Arrhythmia Institute
St. David's Medical Center;
University of Texas
Austin, TX
USA

Charlie Young, MD
Permanente Medical Group
Cardiac Electrophysiology Laboratory
Kaiser-Permanente Medical Center
San Jose, CA
USA

Preface

I was trained to use radiofrequency as the energy source in the ablation of various cardiac arrhythmias more than 20 years ago. This time-honored energy source has been shown to perform well in terms of both efficacy and safety profile. It was not until I encountered my first complication of inadvertent permanent atrioventricular block, in a young patient who underwent catheter ablation for atrioventricular nodal reentrant tachycardia, that I recognized we might need an even better source of energy.

Certainly, catheter cryoablation is not a substitute for radiofrequency ablation. However, in many of the arrhythmic substrates (notably the perinodal area, Koch's triangle, pulmonary vein, coronary sinus, cavotricuspid isthmus, etc.), cryothermy may be considered as the energy source of choice. Unfortunately, there has been a shortage of educational materials in this area. This work thus represents the first book dedicated to the science and practice of catheter cryoablation.

The Practice of Catheter Cryoablation for Cardiac Arrhythmias is purposefully written and organized to update the knowledge base in catheter cryoablation, with the emphasis on "how to perform." We compare cryothermy with radiofrequency energy source in different arrhythmic substrates, and we have also supplemented the textual content with a companion website (www.chancryoablation.com) providing interactive cases and real case videos for selected chapters.

I am sure that this book can benefit all those who are interested in better understanding this relatively new technology and the science behind it. More importantly, this book will serve as an indispensable reference for those who would like to adopt catheter cryoablation in treating patients with different cardiac arrhythmias.

Ngai-Yin Chan, MBBS, FRCP, FACC, FHRS

Acknowledgments

This book is the product of the collective effort of many dedicated people. I would like to thank all the contributing authors, who are all prominent leaders in the field of catheter cryoablation and have found time out of their busy schedules to write the various chapters of the book. I also thank my great colleagues Stephen Choy and Johnny Yuen, who were excellent assistants during my cryoablation procedures. Stephen Cheung, an expert radiologist and a good friend of mine, has to be acknowledged for his contribution of the beautiful reconstructed cardiac CT image that is used on the book cover. Lastly, I have to thank Adam Wang and Perry Tang for their technical support in the preparation of the live cryoablation procedures videos for the companion website.

About the Companion Website

This book is accompanied by a companion website:

www.chancryoablation.com

The website includes:

- Interactive Case Studies to accompany Chapters 2, 4, 5, 6, 7, 8 and 10
- Video clips to illustrate various cryoablation procedures

CHAPTER 1

Biophysical Principles and Properties of Cryoablation

Jo Jo Hai and Hung-Fat Tse

Queen Mary Hospital, The University of Hong Kong, Hong Kong, China

Background

More than 4000 years have passed since the first documented medical use of cooling therapy, when the ancient Egyptian Edwin Smith Papyrus described applying cold compresses made up of figs, honey, and grease to battlefield injuries.[1] Not until 1947 did Hass and Taylor first describe the creation of myocardial lesions using cold energy generated by carbon dioxide as a refrigerant.[2] In contrast to the destructive nature of heat energy, which produces diffuse areas of hemorrhage and necrosis with thrombus formation and aneurysmal dilation, cryoablation involves a unique biophysical process that gives it the distinctive safety and efficacy profile.[3] Cryoablation induces cellular damage mainly via disruption of membranous organelles, such that destruction to the gross myocardial architectures is reduced. Furthermore, cryomapping is feasible as lesions created at a less cool temperature ($>-30\,^{\circ}\mathrm{C}$) are reversible. These potential advantages nurtured the extensive clinical applications of cryoablation in the treatment of cardiac arrhythmias, such as atrioventricular nodal reentrant tachycardia, septal accessory pathways, atrial fibrillation, and ventricular tachycardia, where a high degree of precision is desirable.

Thermodynamics of the cryoablation system

Heat flows from higher temperature to lower temperature zones. Cryoablation destroys tissue by removing heat from it via a probe that is cooled down to freezing temperatures, which has been made feasible by the invention of refrigerants that permit ultra-effective cooling.

Joule–Thompson effect

In the 1850s, James Prescott Joule and William Thomson described the temperature change of a gas when it is forced through a valve and allowed to expand in an insulated environment. Above the inversion temperature, gas molecules move faster. When they collide with each other, kinetic energy is temporarily converted into potential energy. The average distance between molecules increases as gas expands. This results in significantly fewer collisions between molecules, thus lowers the stored

The Practice of Catheter Cryoablation for Cardiac Arrhythmias, First Edition. Edited by Ngai-Yin Chan.
© 2014 John Wiley & Sons, Ltd. Published 2014 by John Wiley & Sons, Ltd.

potential energy. Because the total energy is conserved, there is a parallel increase in the kinetic energy of the gas. Temperature increases.

In contrast, gas molecules move slower at temperatures below the inversion point. The effect of collision-associated energy conversion becomes less important. The average distance between molecules increases when the gas is allowed to expand. The intermolecular attractive forces (van der Waals forces) increase, and so does the stored potential energy. As the total energy is conserved, there is a parallel decrease in the kinetic energy of the gas. Temperature decreases.[4]

Invention of refrigerant
In the 1870s, Carl Paul Gottfried von Linde applied the Joule–Thompson effect to develop the first commercial refrigeration machine. In his original design, liquefied air was first cooled down by a series of heat exchangers, followed by rapid expansion through a nozzle into an isolated chamber, such that the gas rapidly cooled down to freezing temperature. The cold air generated was then coupled with a countercurrent heat exchanger, where ambient air was chilled before expansion began. This further lowered the temperature of the compressed air entering the apparatus, and it increased the efficiency of the machine (Figure 1.1).[5]

According to the principles of the Joule–Thompson effect, only gases with a high inversion temperature can be used as refrigerants. This is because gases with a low inversion temperature under atmospheric pressure, such as hydrogen and helium, warm up rather than cool down during expansion.[6]

Modern cryoablation system
A cryoprobe is a high-pressure, closed-loop gas expansion system. The cryogen travels along the vacuum's central lumen under pressure to the distal electrode, where it is forced through a throttle and rapidly expands to atmospheric pressure. This causes a dramatic drop in the temperature of the metallic tip, so that the heat of tissue in contact with it is rapidly carried away by conduction and convection. The depressurized gas then returns to the console, where it is restored to the liquid state (Figure 1.2).[3,6]

The probe temperature varies with the cryogen used. The most widely used cryogens in surgery are liquid nitrogen, which can attain a temperature as low as −196 °C; and argon gas, which can achieve a temperature as low as −186 °C.[7] Nevertheless, the complex and bulky delivery systems for these agents limit their utility in percutaneous cardiac procedures. To date, only a nitrous oxide–based cryocatheter is commercially available for use by cardiologists, and its lowest achievable temperature is −89.5 °C.[3,7,8]

The minimal temperature and maximal cooling rate occur at the tissue in contact with the metal tip. With increasing distance from the tip, the nadir temperature rises, cooling rates decrease, and

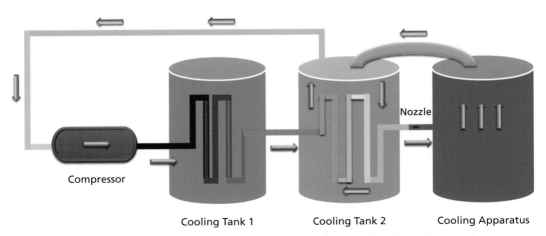

Figure 1.1. Schematic representation of the von Linde refrigerator. The direction of air flow is shown by the arrows.

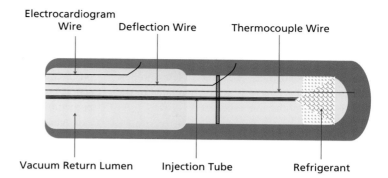

Figure 1.2. Schematic diagram to show the design of the cryoablation probe.

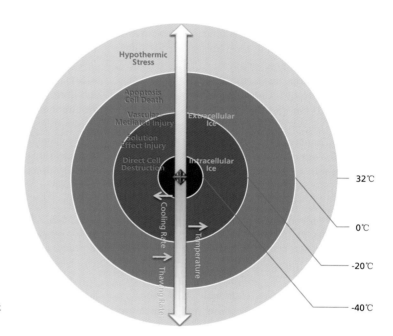

Figure 1.3. Isotherm map of the tip of the catheter electrode of a cryoablation probe (marked by the cross). As shown here, different mechanisms of cell injuries occur at different temperatures.

thawing rates increase. The resultant isotherm map determines the mechanism of injury of those cells lying within each temperature zone, and hence the outcome of the procedure (Figure 1.3).[8]

Mechanisms of injury

Freezing results in both immediate and delayed damage to the targeted tissue. Immediate effects include hypothermic stress and direct cell injury, while delayed consequences are the results of vascular-mediated injury and apoptotic cell death.[5]

Hypothermic stress

When the temperature is lowered to below 32 °C, the membranes of the cells and organelles become less fluid, causing ion pumps to lose their transport capabilities. Electrophysiologically, this is reflected by a decrease in the amplitude of action potential, an increase in its duration, and an extension of the repolarization period. As the temperature continues to decline, metabolism slows, ion imbalances occur, intracellular pH lowers, and adenosine triphosphate levels decrease.[9] Intracellular calcium accumulation secondary to ion pump inactivity and failure of the sarcoplasmic reticulum reuptake mechanism may lead to further free radical generation and cellular disruption.[5] Nevertheless, these effects are entirely transient, provided that the duration of cooling does not exceed a few minutes. The rapidity of recovery is inversely related to the duration of hypothermic exposure.[3]

Direct cell injury

Contrasting the transient effect of hypothermia, ice formation is the basis of permanent cell injury. When the tissue approaches freezing temperature, ice formation begins and results in cryoadhesion. It acts as a "heat sink" by which heat is rapidly extracted from the tissue.[5] With further lowering of temperature, ice crystals form in both extracellular and intracellular compartments.[3,10,11] Water crystallization begins inside the cells (heterogeneous nucleation) at −15 °C, but intracellular ice generally forms (homogeneous nucleation) at temperatures below −40 °C.[11] Besides, intracellular ice formation is more likely to occur under rapid cooling and at the sites where cells are tightly packed, as water cannot diffuse fast enough through the cellular membrane to equilibrate the intracellular and extracellular compartments.[6,8,10] Intracellular ice compresses and deforms the nuclei and cytoplasmic components, induces pore formation in the plasma membranes, and results in permanent dysfunction of the cellular transport systems and leakage of cellular components.[3,6,8,11] All these events lead to irreversible cell damage and ultimately cell death.

Extracellular ice usually forms under moderate freezing temperatures and slower cooling rates.[3,11] The ice crystals sequestrate free water, which increases solute concentration and hence tonicity of the extracellular compartment. Water is withdrawn from the cells along the osmotic gradient, causing cellular dehydration and elevated intracellular solute concentration. As the process continues, these alterations in the internal environment damage intracellular constituents and destabilize the cell membranes. This is termed *solution–effect injury*.[3,6,11]

Cells densely packed in a tissue are subjected to shearing forces generated between ice crystals, which can result in mechanical destruction.[8,11] However, a previous study has shown that membrane integrity was preserved for up to 2 min after thawing, questioning the actual importance of this theoretical effect.[12]

During thawing, extracellular ice melts and results in hypotonicity of the extracellular compartment. Water is shifted back to the intracellular space, causing cell swelling and bursting. It also perpetuates the growth of intracellular ice crystals, exacerbating cell destruction and cell death. This process of recrystallization occurs at temperatures between −40 and −15 °C, predominantly from −25 to −20 °C.[8,9,11]

Delayed cell death

Cooling results in vasoconstriction, which jeopardizes blood flow to the tissue supplied.[11] At −20 to −10 °C, vascular stasis occurs, water crystallizes, and endothelial cell injury ensues.[11,13] When the blood flow restores at the thawing phase, platelets aggregate and form thrombi at the sites of endothelial injury, leading to small vessel occlusion.[11] The resultant ischemia triggers an influx of vasoactive substances that lead to regional hyperemia and tissue edema, and migration of inflammatory cells that clear up cell debris.[4,6,11] The chance of cell survival is minimized, and uniform coagulation necrosis develops.[4,6,8]

Cells that survive the initial freeze and thaw phases may also die from apoptosis in the next few hours to days.[8] This is because cellular injuries, especially damage to the mitochondria, activate caspases, which cleave proteins and cause membrane blebbing, chromatin condensation, genomic fragmentation, and programmed cell death.[8,13] This is particularly important at the peripheral zone of ablation, where temperatures and cooling rates achieved are less likely to be immediately lethal to the cells.

Lesion characteristics

A detailed description of the histological effect of cryoablation has been published elsewhere.[12] In summary, it can be divided into three phases: the immediate postthaw phase, hemorrhagic and inflammatory phase, and replacement fibrosis phase.

Immediate postthaw phase

Within 30 min of thawing, the myocytes become swollen and the myofilaments appear stretched. The

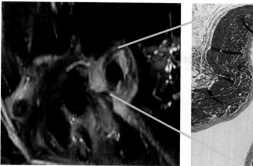
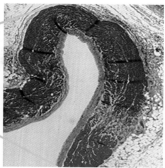

Figure 1.4. Examples of gross (left panel) and histological (right panel) sections show cryoablation lesions after percutaneous cryoablation at the pulmonary vein in a canine. Note the well-demarcated boundary and intact endothelial layer at the site of the cryoablation lesion.

increase in membrane permeability causes mitochondria to swell, which results in oxidation of the endogenous pyridine nucleotides, membrane lipid peroxidation, and enzymatic hydrolysis. This is followed by progressive loss in myofilament structure and irreversible mitochondrial damage.[12]

Hemorrhagic and inflammatory phase

Coagulation necrosis, characterized by hemorrhage, edema, and inflammation, becomes evident at the central part of the lesion within 48 hours after thawing.[12] At the peripheral zone, apoptosis progressively increases and becomes apparent in 8 to 12 hours. At 1 week, infiltrates of inflammatory cells, fibrin and collagen stranding, and capillary ingrowth sharply demarcate the periphery of the lesion.[12] Endothelial layers remain intact, and thrombus formation is uncommon compared with radiofrequency ablation.[14]

Replacement fibrosis phase

Necrotic tissue is largely cleared up by the end of the fourth week. The lesion now consists mainly of dense collagen fibers and fat infiltration, with new blood vessels reestablishing at the periphery. Healing continues for 3 months until a small, fibrotic scar with an intact endothelial layer and a well-demarcated boundary is formed (Figure 1.4).

Factors affecting cryoablation efficacy

The success of cryoablation depends on its ability to deliver a lethal condition to the targeted cells. Although it is more clinically relevant to define it by the completeness of tissue destruction or ablation outcomes, most of the literature has compared only the size of cryolesions produced under different conditions. A summary of our current knowledge

in the optimal freezing parameters is discussed in this section.

Tissue temperature

A lower temperature probe creates a deeper lesion, with each $10\,°C$ decrease in the nadir temperature increasing the depth of lesion by $0.4\,mm$.[3] Although many experiments have shown that extensive damage occurs between -30 and $-20\,°C$, destruction may be incomplete for some types of tissue.[7,8,11] In particular, muscle cells including cardiomyocytes are very sensitive to freezing injury, while cancer cells appear to be much more resistant.[8,11] Generally speaking, a nadir temperature below $-40\,°C$ is preferred, as this is the temperature required to produce direct cell injury through lethal intracellular ice formation, and experiments have confirmed that almost all cell types died after rapid cooling to $-40\,°C$.[6]

Cooling rate

Studies have shown that intracellular ice tends to form with rapid freezing. This is because a slow cooling rate increases the duration of exposure of the cells to a higher temperature environment, where extracellular ice is preferentially formed. This in turn causes cellular dehydration and elevated solute concentration, and lowers the intracellular freezing temperature. These alterations in the internal environment hamper the formation of intracellular ice crystals, making cellular destruction less effective.[6]

In reality, rapid freezing (i.e. more than $-50\,°C$ per min) occurs only at the cryotip. At about $1\,cm$ from the tip, the cooling rate rapidly drops to -10 to $-20\,°C$ per min.[11] While affecting the mode of cellular injury, in vivo experiments, however, have not shown that cooling rate per second is a primary determinant of ablation outcomes.[7,11]

Duration of freezing

The duration of freezing is probably unimportant at the cryotip (where the tissue temperature rapidly reaches −50 °C), as all intracellular water is frozen immediately.[7,11] However, as the cooling effect reduces across the ablation zone, a large portion of tissue will only attain a lower nadir temperature over a longer period of time. Prolongation of freezing not only provides time for the peripheral tissue to reach its lowest achievable temperature such that lethal ice may form, but also increases cell death through solution–effect injury and water recrystallization.[7,11] Indeed, prior studies have shown that 5 min of freezing created significantly larger and deeper cryolesions when compared to 2.5 min of freezing,[15] although the optimal freezing duration for each tissue type has not yet been clearly defined.

Thawing rate

Studies have shown that time to electrode rewarming predicts lesion size.[16] It is thought that prolonged rewarming increases time for cell damage by solution–effect injury and water recrystallization, as both occur during tissue thawing.[7,8,11] In practice, this can be done by passive rewarming.

Freeze-thaw cycles

Early experiments have shown that by repeating the freeze-thaw cycle, both the size of the lesion and the extent of necrosis are increased. This is because thermal conduction is enhanced by the initial cellular breakdown, such that subsequent cycles may lead to more substantial tissue destruction.[7,8] This is especially critical at the peripheral zone of ablation, where the nadir temperature is higher and cell damage tends to be incomplete.

Although the development of newer cryoablation technology that enables much a lower freezing temperature and faster cooling rate may alter the benefit of repeating the freeze-thaw cycle,[3] it is probably still advisable in the treatment of malignancy, where complete tissue destruction is of utmost importance.[8]

Blood flow

Blood flow is a heat source that increases the difficulty of freezing by altering the cooling rate, thawing rate, and lowest attainable temperature.[17] Experimentation has shown that by lowering the

blood flow velocity, lesion volume increases.[16,18,19] For this reason, cryoablation is particularly effective when used in low-flow regions such as areas with trabeculations.

Size of catheter tip

Studies have shown that both surface area and volume of cryolesions increase with the size of the catheter tip.[19,20] Possible explanations include an increase in the amount of tissue in direct contact with the cryotip, and a difference in tip-to-tissue contact angles. Nevertheless, lesion depth remains independent of the size of catheter used.

Electrode orientation

In contrast to radiofrequency ablation, in cryoablation significantly larger lesions are created using horizontal rather than vertical catheter tip-to-tissue orientation, probably due to the reduction in parts of the electrode exposed to the warming effect of the blood pool.[15,16,18] Again, only surface dimensions, but not depth of the lesions, are found to be affected.

Contact pressure

Although it is commonly believed that constant contact pressure is not necessary during cryoablation as the ice formed at the catheter tip acts as a reliable thermal conductor, studies have consistently proved that better tissue contact improves lesion sizes and is desirable.[16,18,19]

Conclusion

With its unique mechanism of tissue injury, cryoenergy has demonstrated various advantages over hyperthermic destruction: catheter stability can be improved by cryoadhesion formed from extracellular ice; ablation of vital structures can be prevented by cryomapping, as cell damage is largely reversible at the ablation onset; and thromboembolism can be avoided due to the lack of thrombus formation. All these factors allow cryoablation to gain favor for use among populations and procedures that desire high safety profiles. Nevertheless, optimal lesion creation still depends on catheter design and on freezing parameters, including duration, repeated freeze-thaw cycles, tissue contact, as well as the local warming effect from the surrounding blood flow. With better defined catheters and freezing parameters based on ablation outcomes, and the development of new cryogens and delivery systems, the safety and efficacy profiles of cryoablation will continue to improve. It is foreseeable that the application of cryoablation in the treatment of cardiac arrhythmias will continue to expand in the future.

References

1. Breasted JH. The Edwin Smith Surgical Papyrus. Chicago: University of Chicago Press; 1980.
2. Hass GM, Taylor CB. A quantitative hypothermal method for production of local injury to tissue. Federation Proc. 1947;6:393.
3. Khairy P, Dubuc M. Transcatheter cryoablation part I: preclinical experience. PACE. 2008;31:112–20.
4. Joule JP, Thompson W. On the thermal effects of fluids in motion (part I). Phil Trans Royal Soc London. 1853;143:357–66.
5. Snyder KK, Baust JG, Baust JM, et al. Cryoablation of cardiac arrhythmias. Philadelphia, PA: Elsevier/Saunders; 2011.
6. Erinjeri JP, Clark TW. Cryoablation: mechanism of action and devices. JVIR. 2010;21(8 Suppl.):S187–91.
7. Gage AA, Baust JM, Baust JG. Experimental cryosurgery investigations in vivo. Cryobiology. 2009;59:229–43.
8. Baust JG, Gage AA. The molecular basis of cryosurgery. BJU Intl. 2005;95:1187–91.
9. Baust J, Gage AA, Ma H, et al. Minimally invasive cryosurgery – technological advances. Cryobiology. 1997;34:373–84.
10. Rubinsky B. Cryosurgery. Ann Rev Biomed Eng. 2000;2:157–87.
11. Gage AA, Baust J. Mechanisms of tissue injury in cryosurgery. Cryobiology. 1998;37:171–86.
12. Lustgarten DL, Keane D, Ruskin J. Cryothermal ablation: mechanism of tissue injury and current experience in the treatment of tachyarrhythmias. Prog Cardiovasc Dis. 1999;41:481–98.
13. Finelli A, Rewcastle JC, Jewett MA. Cryotherapy and radiofrequency ablation: pathophysiologic basis and laboratory studies. Curr Opin Urol. 2003;13:187–91.
14. Khairy P, Chauvet P, Lehmann J, et al. Lower incidence of thrombus formation with cryoenergy versus radiofrequency catheter ablation. Circulation. 2003;107:2045–50.
15. Tse HF, Ripley KL, Lee KL, et al. Effects of temporal application parameters on lesion dimensions during transvenous catheter cryoablation. J Cardiovasc Electrophysiol. 2005;16:201–4.
16. Parvez B, Goldberg SM, Pathak V, et al. Time to electrode rewarming after cryoablation predicts lesion size. J Cardiovasc Electrophysiol. 2007;18:845–8.
17. Zhao G, Zhang HF, Guo XJ, et al. Effect of blood flow and metabolism on multidimensional heat transfer during cryosurgery. Med Eng Phys. 2007;29:205–15.
18. Parvez B, Pathak V, Schubert CM, et al. Comparison of lesion sizes produced by cryoablation and open irrigation radiofrequency ablation catheters. J Cardiovasc Electrophysiol. 2008;19:528–34.
19. Wood MA, Parvez B, Ellenbogen AL, et al. Determinants of lesion sizes and tissue temperatures during catheter cryoablation. PACE. 2007;30:644–54.
20. Khairy P, Rivard L, Guerra PG, et al. Morphometric ablation lesion characteristics comparing 4, 6, and 8 mm electrode-tip cryocatheters. J Cardiovasc Electrophysiol. 2008;19:1203–7.

CHAPTER 2

Catheter Cryoablation for Pediatric Arrhythmias

Kathryn K. Collins[1] and George F. Van Hare[2]

[1]University of Colorado and Children's Hospital Colorado, Aurora, CO, USA
[2]Washington University School of Medicine and St. Louis Children's Hospital, St. Louis, MO, USA

Introduction

In pediatric patients with otherwise normal heart structure, the most commonly encountered tachyarrhythmias are accessory pathway–mediated tachycardia and atrioventricular nodal reentrant tachycardia (AVNRT). Catheter ablation techniques for these tachyarrhythmias are generally similar to those utilized in adult patients, but they are modified for patient size. Also notable is that the risk–benefit ratio in pediatric ablations favors a focus on safety. A complication such as atrioventricular block requiring a pacemaker would cause significant morbidity to an otherwise healthy child. While radiofrequency catheter ablation has been shown to have a high success rate and limited complications in a pediatric population,[1–4] cryoablation continues to be utilized in pediatrics primarily because of the safety of cryoablation around structures such as the atrioventricular node.[5–29] This chapter will review cryoablation techniques, clinical out-comes, and current utilization of cryoablation for tachyarrhythmias in a pediatric population.

Cryoablation in immature myocardium – animal studies

There has always been concern about the effects of ablation on the immature myocardium. A prior report had shown that radiofrequency ablation lesions placed in fetal lambs showed increasing size of the lesion.[30] A study for cryoablation in piglets has shown that cryoablation lesions in immature atrial and ventricular myocardium enlarge to a similar extent compared to those caused by radiofrequency ablation.[31] In contrast, atrioventricular groove lesion volumes do not increase significantly with either energy modality.[31] Similarly, a separate study, again in piglets, showed no evidence of coronary artery obstruction or intimal plaque formation early or late after cryoenergy application.[32] Thus, with cryoablation, there is still concern for

---

lesion enlargement in the immature myocardium. There is less concern for potential effects on the coronary arteries.

Transcatheter cryoablation technique for the treatment of tachyarrhythmias in pediatrics

Electrophysiology study

The electrophysiology study is conducted in a similar fashion for radiofrequency ablation or cryoablation procedures. Antiarrhythmic medications are usually discontinued for at least five half-lives before the procedure. Procedures are conducted under general anesthesia or intravenous moderate or deep sedation. Electrode catheters are placed in the high right atrium, the His bundle position, the right ventricular apex, and the coronary sinus. Standard atrial and ventricular pacing protocols are then conducted to document the arrhythmia mechanism. If no arrhythmia is inducible, isoproterenol is administered and the pacing protocol is repeated.

Cryoablation technique – general aspects

The cryoablation catheter (Cryocath Technologies, Canada) is advanced from the femoral vein into the heart. The catheters are 7 French size and generally move easily through 7 or 8 French-sized sheaths. The catheters have 4 mm, 6 mm, or 8 mm tip sizes and are available in small, medium, and large curves. The choice of catheter tip size is at the discretion of the electrophysiologist. In the United States, the 4 mm tip is the only catheter that currently has regulatory approval for test lesions of cryomapping (discussed in this chapter). The 6 mm tip size is currently the most commonly utilized catheter, with the 4 mm used for younger patients and the 8 mm tip utilized for larger patents. The catheters are relatively stiff in comparison to available radiofrequency catheters. When placed into the heart and onto the atrioventricular groove, our practice has been to advance the catheter by first turning away from the septum in order to avoid mechanical injury to atrioventricular conduction, related to stiffness of the catheter. The catheter is then placed at the site chosen for ablation – on the atrioventricular groove for accessory pathways or in the area of the slow atrioventricular nodal pathway for AVNRT. Cryoenergy is then applied.

Cryomapping is conducted by freezing to a set point, typically −30 or −40 °C, for a maximum of 1 min, at which time an ice ball forms at the tip of the catheter. The catheter is securely adhered to the myocardium, and due to the engineering of the conductors, intracardiac signals are not available from the catheter tip during the lesion. At this temperature, one can assess for the desired effect (e.g., loss of accessory pathway activity) as well as monitor for continued normal atrioventricular nodal conduction. If the desired effect is seen without changes to the normal conduction, then *cryoablation* is conducted by freezing to a set point of −70 or −80 °C for a total of 4 min. With the 6 mm or 8 mm catheter tip, "fast mapping" is utilized, which translates to monitoring for the desired effect as the cryoablation catheter is frozen to the minimum temperature of −80 °C. It is important to maintain constant monitoring of atrioventricular nodal conduction throughout the entire cryoablation lesion, as deterioration in atrioventricular node conduction can occur late in a cryoablation lesion. Also, cryomapping locations that are deemed safe may show changes in atrioventricular nodal conduction with cryoablation at the same location.[33] If interference with normal atrioventricular conduction is evident, cryoablation should be immediately terminated and the tissue allowed to rewarm. Reliably, if this is done, the effect of cryoablation is still reversible. If the cryoablation catheter is at the precise location for successful ablation, cryoenergy is continued for a 4 min application or longer. Many clinicians advocate a "freeze-thaw-freeze" cycle in order to form a deeper, more permanent cryoablation lesion. Others support lengthier cryoablation lesions (approximately 7 min) and the placement of an extra cryoapplication at the successful site as a means of potentially improving efficacy.[34] The relative importance of these different approaches has not been carefully studied.

Cryoablation catheters may be utilized with long sheaths for catheter stability, which may allow a more precise tip localization prior to onset of cryoadhesion, after which there should be no possibility of catheter dislodgement. Likewise, cryomapping and cryoablation lesions may be placed without the chance for catheter dislodgement either during tachycardia or with the infusion of isoproterenol. In patients who are under general anesthesia, controlled ventilation can also be utilized at the initiation of a cryothermal lesion until the catheter adheres to the myocardium.

Cryoablation technique for AVNRT

As with the radiofrequency ablation approach to AVNRT, the cryoablation catheter is placed in the area of the slow atrioventricular nodal pathway by an anatomic and electrophysiologic approach. Cryomapping and cryoablation lesions are placed in sinus rhythm with simultaneous monitoring for normal atrioventricular nodal conduction. Because of catheter adherence to the myocardium during a cryoablation lesion, cryomapping or cryoablation lesions can also be placed in sinus tachycardia during isoproterenol infusion or during sustained atrioventricular nodal reentry. Our approach in the laboratory is to start low in the septum, and place a cryoablation lesion. After 1 min of the cryoablation lesion formation, atrial pacing is conducted to evaluate for lack of tachycardia inducibility, change in Wenckebach cycle length, or change in response to A1A2 pacing. If there is a change in one of these parameters, then a full 4 min lesion is placed at this location. We then place 3–4 more cryoablation lesions around this level (Figure 2.1a and 2.1b). Retesting is carried out during these ablation lesions, then after all 4–5 lesions are placed. Several modifications to the cryoablation technique have been reported to improve outcomes for AVNRT ablation, and they include increase in number of cryoablation lesions,[34] longer duration of cryoablation lesions,[34] linear ablation lesions,[21] and use of the larger 8 mm tip cryoablation catheter.[6] Finally, it should be noted that the delivery of cryotherapy during sustained AVNRT is a reasonable strategy, as cryoadhesion eliminates the possibility of catheter dislodgement with sudden termination.

The standard procedural endpoint for cryoablation of AVNRT is for no further inducible tachycardia post cryoablation. Unlike the case with radiofrequency applications for posterior atrioventricular nodal modification, cryoablation does not produce accelerated junctional rhythm, and thus this proxy for successful ablation is not feasible with cryoablation. Other criteria for success, such as loss of dual atrioventricular nodal physiology (a $\geq$ 50 msec increase in A2H2 with a 10 msec decrease in A1A2 pacing) or loss of sustained slow pathway conduction (PR $\geq$ RR during atrial overdrive pacing), can be monitored.[25] In our labora-

tory, the most significant pre- versus postcryoablation findings were a reduction in the finding of PR $\geq$ RR during atrial overdrive pacing and a decrease in the maximal AH interval with atrial pacing.[25] Another technique described is monitoring of the atrioventricular nodal fast pathway refractory period during cryoablation.[35] With single atrial extrastimulus pacing (A1A2) during successful cryoablation lesions, there was prolongation of the AV nodal fast pathway effective refractory period by $\geq$20 msec that was not evident at unsuccessful cryoablation sites. In practice, the endpoint of the procedure needs to be tailored to the individual patient's arrhythmia burden, the patient's size and other clinical parameters, as well as the pre-ablation electrophysiologic findings.

Cryoablation technique for ablation of accessory pathways

As with radiofrequency ablation, the cryoablation catheter is placed on the atrioventricular groove at the site of the accessory pathway as determined by standard mapping techniques. The utilization of other three-dimensional mapping systems can also be useful. The cryoablation catheter is maneuvered to the precise location of the pathway, and cryoablation (with or without cryomapping) is carried out. With sites near normal conduction tissue, monitoring should continue throughout the entire cryoablation lesion, observing for the desired effect of loss of accessory pathway and for any changes to atrioventricular nodal conduction. If no change to accessory pathway activity is evident, the lesion is terminated and another location for ablation is sought. Time to effect of loss of accessory pathway conduction of >10 sec has been associated with recurrence of accessory pathway conduction and subsequent recurrent tachycardia (Figure 2.2a and 2.2b).[36,37]

Outcomes of cryoablation in pediatrics

Outcomes of cryoablation for pediatric AVNRT

Multiple manuscripts have been published on the outcomes of cryoablation for AVNRT in a pediatric population (Table 2.1).[9–15,18–21,25–27,29,34–35] In general, outcomes for cryoablation are nearing those for radiofrequency ablation, although with a higher chance of arrhythmia recurrence. For

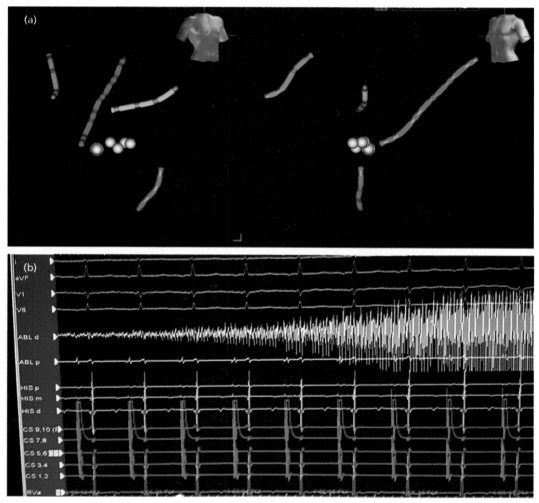

Figure 2.1. (a) Images of a cryoablation procedure for pediatric atrioventricular nodal reentrant tachycardia (AVNRT). Images are from the Ensite Velocity system (St. Jude Medical, MN, United States). Views are shown in 60° right anterior oblique (RAO) and 30° left anterior oblique (LAO) projections. Catheters are as follows: high right atrial (blue), decapolar within the coronary sinus (green), His bundle electrode catheter (yellow), and right ventricular apical catheter (red). The cryoablation catheter is not shown. A linear cryoablation line was created in the posterior septal space. Round white dots represent 4 min cryoablation lesions. (b) Surface and intracardiac electrograms during an application of cryoablation for AVNRT. Typically, lesions are placed in normal sinus rhythm or in atrial paced rhythm (as presented here). The intracardiac signal on the cryoablation catheter (ABL d) shows initial signals of a small "A" electrogram with a larger "V" electrogram. Once temperatures of about −30 °C are reached, the ice ball forms at the catheter tip, and there is loss of signal on the distal electrodes of the ablation catheter. Of note, there usually is no accelerated junctional rhythm seen with a posterior node modification with cryoablation. The timing for AH is monitored throughout the 4 min cryoablation lesion. II, III, aVF, V1: surface electrocardiographic leads; Abl d: ablation distal; Abl p: ablation proximal; CS: coronary sinus; HIS: catheter placed near the His bundle; RV a: right ventricular apex.

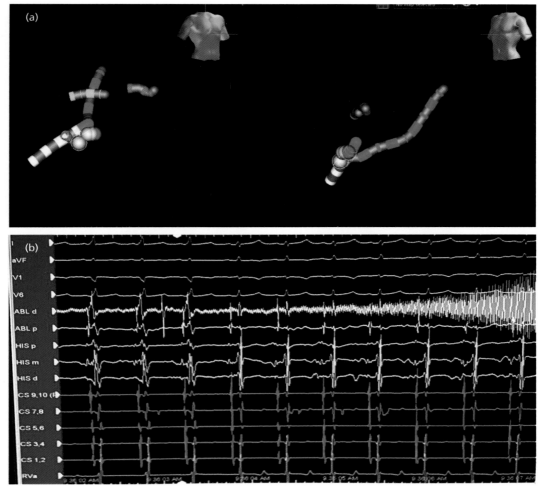

Figure 2.2. (a) Images of a cryoablation procedure for a pediatric patient with a right posterior septal accessory pathway. Images are from the Ensite Velocity system (St. Jude Medical, MN, United States). Views are shown in 60° right anterior oblique (RAO) and 30° left anterior oblique (LAO) projections. Catheters are as follows: decapolar within the coronary sinus (green), His bundle electrode catheter (yellow), right ventricular apical catheter (red), and cryoablation catheter (white with green tip). Because of small patient size, a decapolar catheter was utilized for the His bundle and right ventricular locations. A round green dot depicts the location of the successful cryoablation lesion. Round white dots represent 4 min "insurance" cryoablation lesions. (b) Surface and intracardiac electrograms during an application of cryoablation for right posterior accessory pathway that conducted both antegradely and retrogradely. Mapping and ablation were conducted in pre-excited sinus rhythm. The intracardiac signal on the cryoablation catheter (ABL d) shows fused "A" and "V" electrograms. Once temperatures of about −30 °C are reached, the ice ball forms at the catheter tip, and there is loss of signal on the distal electrodes of the ablation catheter. With this cryomapping, there is successful loss of the antegrade accessory pathway conduction on the fourth beat on the screen, prior to the ice ball formation. II, III, aVF, V1: surface electrocardiographic leads; Abl d: ablation distal; Abl p: ablation proximal; CS: coronary sinus; HIS: catheter placed near the His bundle; RV a: right ventricular apex.

Table 2.1. Clinical outcomes for cryoablation of AVNRT in pediatric patients

Cryoablation	n	Initial success (%)	Recurrence (%)
Kirsh et al. (2005)[15]	30	83	9–14
Miyazaki et al. (2005)[11]	22	96	5
Kriebel et al. (2005)[14]	13	85	0
Drago et al. (2005)[20]	14	93	23
Drago et al. (2006)[34]	29	97	7
Papez et al. (2006)[9]	53	94	12
Collins et al. (2006)[26]	55	98	8
Chanani et al. (2008)[27]	154	95	14
Avari et al. (2008)[29]	38	97	2
Papagiannis et al. (2010)[10]	20	90	28
Silver et al. (2010)[6]	52	87	0
Czosek et al. (2010)[21]	62	94	3
Drago et al. (2010)[19]	64	97	7
LaPage et al. (2010)[12]	73	96	7
Emmel et al. (2011)[18]	30	90	19

radiofrequency ablation for AVNRT, procedural outcomes are reported as 95–100% successful, with arrhythmia recurrence rates at 2–6%. For cryoablation, procedural outcomes have shown 87–98% success if one dismisses the earlier literature as part of the physician learning curve for utilizing cryoablation. The AVNRT recurrence rate has been reported with a range of 0–33%. In some of the larger series, AVNRT recurrence rates for cryoablation are reported as 0–7%, which nears that of radiofrequency ablation. There is a large variability in reported outcomes, which is possibly secondary to the single-center aspect of the published literature and the relatively small sample sizes.

For those patients with AVNRT recurrences who return to the laboratory for a subsequent ablation attempt, the current trend is to utilize radiofrequency ablation.[23] However, some centers continue to have a preference for cryoablation for a second attempt, perhaps utilizing one of the modifications in technique to improve long-term success.

A specific subset of AVNRT patients has documented narrow complex tachycardia that is reentrant in nature, but when they are assessed in the laboratory, there is no evidence of an accessory pathway and no inducible tachycardia. These patients are considered to have "presumed AVNRT." Prior reports suggest that radiofrequency applications for AV nodal slow pathway modification can lead to permanent cure in these patients. In a manuscript currently submitted for publication, we evaluated 13 patients with presumed AVNRT who underwent cryoablation. The endpoint utilized for cryoablation in this series was largely evidence of sustained slow pathway conduction as evidenced by PR ≥ RR. In this series of patients, there was an arrhythmia recurrence rate of 23%. Cryoablation can be utilized in this patient group, but a clearer ablation endpoint needs to be established for long-term cure.

Within the studies for cryoablation for AVNRT, there has been no permanent atrioventricular block. Transient atrioventricular block has been reported, but all resolved shortly after rewarming of the cardiac tissue. In comparison, there is a 0–2% risk of permanent atrioventricular block with radiofrequency ablation for AVNRT in similar patient populations.[1]

Outcomes of cryoablation of accessory pathway ablation in pediatrics

The published reports for cryoablation of accessory pathway ablation in children are largely single-center experiences with relatively small patient sample sizes (Table 2.2).[5,9,11,13–18,28,34,36–37] The success rates for cryoablation of accessory pathways in pediatrics are disappointing, with initial success rates reported as 60–100% and recurrence

Table 2.2. Clinical outcomes of cryoablation for accessory pathway–mediated tachycardia in pediatrics

Cryoablation	n	Initial success (%)	Recurrence (%)
Gaita et al. (2004)[17]	4	100	25
Kirsh et al. (2005)[15]	30	60	9–14
Miyazaki et al. (2005) [11]	8	63	40
Drago et al. (2005)[20]	12	92	36
Kriebel et al. (2005)[15]	19	68	23
Bar-Cohen et al. (2006)[28]	35	78	45
Drago et al. (2006)[34]	21	95	25
Papez et al. (2006)[9]	20	85	12
Tuzcu (2007)[5]	39	73	24
Kaltman et al. (2008)[36]	25	96	—
Drago et al. (2009)[37]	31	97	20
Gist et al. (2009)[16]	29	97	4
Emmel et al. (2011)[18]	6	100	33

rates of 4–45%. This wide range of success and recurrence rates likely reflects the variability in the location and type of targeted accessory pathways and the learning curve and experience of each center. Practice patterns (discussed in the "Practice Trends in Pediatric Cryoablation" section) are such that pediatric electrophysiologists largely utilize cryoablation only for substrates near the atrioventricular node and continue to have a preference for radiofrequency ablation for accessory pathways away from the normal conduction. For paraHisian substrates, some of the accessory pathways would have been deemed too close to the normal conduction to attempt radiofrequency ablation, but because of the safety profile an attempt with cryoablation was considered acceptable. The electrophysiologist would still be cautious around the atrioventricular node and not place insurance lesions or freeze-thaw-freeze lesions in order to assure no damage to the atrioventricular node. Recurrences in this group have been associated with younger patient age and midseptal accessory pathway location.[28]

The outcome data also reflect a relatively high proportion of right free wall accessory pathways that are known to have a higher arrhythmia recurrence rate with radiofrequency ablation techniques. Anecdotally, there is some thought that cryoablation may be beneficial for right-sided accessory pathways, where it is difficult to maneuver a standard radiofrequency ablation catheter to remain on the atrioventricular groove; since the cryoablation catheter "grabs" the tissue when the ice ball forms, constant contact with the pathway location is improved. However, outcome data (Table 2.2) do not support this hypothesis. One report specifically focused on cryoablation within the coronary sinus, and for this particular substrate, there is a low initial success rate and high arrhythmia recurrence rate.[24] For the substrate of permanent junctional reciprocating tachycardia, the patient numbers are small, but the initial success rate is reported as 100%.[17,28] One center has published outcomes of cryoablation for left-sided accessory pathways, with good initial and midterm outcomes.[16]

As with AVNRT ablation, there has been no reported permanent atrioventricular block as a result of cryoablation.

Cryoablation for other substrates

Limited data are available for cryoablation with other arrhythmia substrates. There are several case reports of successful cryoablation for non-postoperative junctional ectopic tachycardia (JET) without damage to atrioventricular nodal function.[7,38] One multicenter study on the clinical outcome of JET described radiofrequency ablation and cryoablation therapy for JET.[22] In this series, radiofrequency ablation (n = 17) had an 82% success rate, a 14% recurrence rate, and an 18%

complication rate for complete atrioventricular block. Cryoablation had an 85% success rate, a 13% recurrence rate, and no atrioventricular block.

Cryoablation for ectopic atrial tachycardia and ventricular tachyarrhythmias is much less common.[15,39]

Cryoablation in congenital heart disease

There have been published case reports of the use of cryoablation for arrhythmias arising near the normal conduction system in patients with congenital heart disease.[8,40] The potential benefit of cryoablation in congenital heart disease would be for those patients in whom the normal conduction system is displaced from its usual anatomic location. Because of the reversible nature of temporary cryoablation lesions, cryoablation could be utilized safely in these substrates without risk of damaging the conduction system. Figure 2.3 depicts a cryoablation procedure for AVNRT in a patient with D-transposition of the great arteries status post a

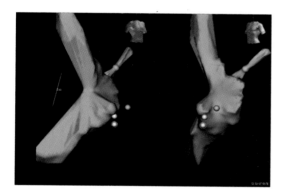

Figure 2.3. Images of a cryoablation procedure for atrioventricular nodal reentrant tachycardia (AVNRT) in a patient with D-transposition of the great arteries status post a Mustard palliation. Images are from the Ensite Velocity system (St. Jude Medical, MN, United States). Views are shown in 60° right anterior oblique (RAO) and 30° left anterior oblique (LAO) projections. Catheters are as follows: the esophageal catheter is marked and was utilized for a system reference. The round yellow dot represents the location where a His bundle electrogram was documented. Round white dots represent 4 min cryoablation lesions that successfully cured the patient from the AVNRT. The catheter approach for this ablation was transbaffle leak to the pulmonary venous atrium.

Mustard ablation. Cryoablation was carried out through a baffle leak.[40]

Practice trends in pediatric cryoablation

Because of the potential safety aspects of cryoablation, many pediatric electrophysiologists readily adopted this technique when it became commercially available. Initially, cryoablation was utilized for all arrhythmia substrates, including AVNRT, accessory pathways on the right or left side, ectopic atrial tachycardias, and ventricular tachycardia. Over the following years and after a "learning curve" for physicians, further studies showed that the recurrence rates for almost all arrhythmia substrates were higher when compared to clinical outcomes for radiofrequency ablation of the same substrates. Most pediatric electrophysiologists then primarily utilized cryoablation for those substrates near the normal conduction system, where, on balance, one would accept a slightly higher chance of arrhythmia recurrence for improved safety and limited risk of development of atrioventricular block. Almost all centers abandoned cryoablation for left-sided accessory pathways, except for one center that championed the technique. In a 2010 survey of pediatric electrophysiologists, 50% utilized cryoablation as the first-line technique for the substrate of AVNRT and 94% utilized it for substrates along the septum that would be considered at high risk for atrioventricular block.[23] The most common reason for choosing radiofrequency over cryoablation was the reported higher arrhythmia recurrence rates with cryoablation.

Cryoablation catheters, as described in this chapter, are relatively stiff and have less maneuverability than standard radiofrequency catheters. Some have questioned their use in younger patients with smaller heart sizes. A multicenter report reviewed the outcome of cryoablation in a pediatric population with weight < 15 kg or age < 5 years.[13] The conclusion of this report was that cryoablation was safe and efficacious for this patient population.

Another consideration for use of cryoablation that was not addressed in the survey is the emerging era of nonfluoroscopic imaging for invasive electrophysiology study and ablation.[41] Perhaps the safety profile of cryoablation allows complete nonfluoroscopic approaches without significant concern for inadvertent atrioventricular block.

Interactive Case Studies related to this chapter can be found at this book's companion website, at **www.chancryoablation.com**

References

1. Van Hare GF, Javitz H, Carmelli D, *et al.* Prospective assessment after pediatric cardiac ablation: demographics, medical profiles, and initial outcomes. J Cardiovasc Electrophysiol. 2004;15:759–70.

2. Van Hare GF, Javitz H, Carmelli D, *et al.* Prospective assessment after pediatric cardiac ablation: recurrence at 1 year after initially successful ablation of supraventricular tachycardia. Heart Rhythm. 2004; 1:188–96.

3. Van Hare GF, Carmelli D, Smith WM, *et al.* Prospective assessment after pediatric cardiac ablation: design and implementation of the multicenter study. Pacing Clin Electrophysiol. 2002;25:332–41.

4. Fishberger SB, Whalen R, Zahn EM, *et al.* Radiofrequency ablation of pediatric AV nodal reentrant tachycardia during the ice age: a single center experience in the cryoablation era. Pacing Clin Electrophysiol. 2010;33:6–10.

5. Tuzcu V. Cryoablation of accessory pathways in children. Pacing Clin Electrophysiol. 2007;30:1129–35.

6. Silver ES, Silva JN, Ceresnak SR, *et al.* Cryoablation with an 8-mm tip catheter for pediatric atrioventricular nodal reentrant tachycardia is safe and efficacious with a low incidence of recurrence. Pacing Clin Electrophysiol. 2010;33:681–6.

7. Shah MJ, Wieand T, Vetter VL. Cryoablation of congenital familial ectopic tachycardia with preservation of atrioventricular nodal function in an infant. J Cardiovasc Electrophysiol. 2007;18:773–6.

8. Rausch CM, Runciman M, Collins KK. Cryothermal catheter ablation of atrioventricular nodal reentrant tachycardia in a pediatric patient after atrioventricular canal repair. Congenit Heart Dis. 2010;5:66–9.

9. Papez AL, Al-Ahdab M, Dick M, 2nd, *et al.* Transcatheter cryotherapy for the treatment of supraventricular tachyarrhythmias in children: a single center experience. J Interv Card Electrophysiol. 2006;15: 191–6.

10. Papagiannis J, Papadopoulou K, Rammos S, *et al.* Cryoablation versus radiofrequency ablation for atrioventricular nodal reentrant tachycardia in children: long-term results. Hellenic J Cardiol. 2010;51: 122–6.

11. Miyazaki A, Blaufox AD, Fairbrother DL, *et al.* Cryoablation for septal tachycardia substrates in pediatric

12. LaPage MJ, Saul JP, Reed JH. Long-term outcomes for cryoablation of pediatric patients with atrioventricular nodal reentrant tachycardia. Am J Cardiol. 2010;105:1118–21.

13. LaPage MJ, Reed JH, Collins KK, *et al.* Safety and results of cryoablation in patients <5 years old and/ or <15 kilograms. Am J Cardiol. 2011;108:565–71.

14. Kriebel T, Broistedt C, Kroll M, *et al.* Efficacy and safety of cryoenergy in the ablation of atrioventricular reentrant tachycardia substrates in children and adolescents. J Cardiovasc Electrophysiol. 2005;16:960–6.

15. Kirsh JA, Gross GJ, O'Connor S, *et al.* Transcatheter cryoablation of tachyarrhythmias in children: initial experience from an international registry. J Am Coll Cardiol. 2005;45:133–6.

16. Gist KM, Bockoven JR, Lane J, *et al.* Acute success of cryoablation of left-sided accessory pathways: a single institution study. J Cardiovasc Electrophysiol. 2009;20:637–42.

17. Gaita F, Montefusco A, Riccardi R, *et al.* Cryoenergy catheter ablation: a new technique for treatment of permanent junctional reciprocating tachycardia in children. J Cardiovasc Electrophysiol. 2004;15: 263–8.

18. Emmel M, Sreeram N, Khalil M, *et al.* Cryoenergy for the ablation of arrhythmogenic paraseptal substrates in children and adolescents with heart rhythm disorders. Dtsch Med Wochenschr. 2011;136:2187–91.

19. Drago F, Russo MS, Silvetti MS, *et al.* Cryoablation of typical atrioventricular nodal reentrant tachycardia in children: six years' experience and follow-up in a single center. Pacing Clin Electrophysiol. 2010;33: 475–81.

20. Drago F, De Santis A, Grutter G, *et al.* Transvenous cryothermal catheter ablation of re-entry circuit located near the atrioventricular junction in pediatric patients: efficacy, safety, and midterm follow-up. J Am Coll Cardiol. 2005;45:1096–103.

21. Czosek RJ, Anderson J, Marino BS, *et al.* Linear lesion cryoablation for the treatment of atrioventricular nodal re-entry tachycardia in pediatrics and young adults. Pacing Clin Electrophysiol. 2010;33: 1304–11.

22. Collins KK, Van Hare GF, Kertesz NJ, *et al.* Pediatric nonpost-operative junctional ectopic tachycardia medical management and interventional therapies. J Am Coll Cardiol. 2009;53:690–7.

23. Collins KK, Schaffer MS. Use of cryoablation for treatment of tachyarrhythmias in 2010: survey of current practices of pediatric electrophysiologists. Pacing Clin Electrophysiol. 2011;34:304–8.

24. Collins KK, Rhee EK, Kirsh JA, *et al.* Cryoablation of accessory pathways in the coronary sinus in young

patients: a multicenter study from the Pediatric and Congenital Electrophysiology Society's Working Group on Cryoablation. J Cardiovasc Electrophysiol. 2007;18:592–7.

25. Collins KK, Dubin AM, Chiesa NA, et al. Cryoablation in pediatric atrioventricular nodal reentry: electrophysiologic effects on atrioventricular nodal conduction. Heart Rhythm. 2006;3:557–63.

26. Collins KK, Dubin AM, Chiesa NA, et al. Cryoablation versus radiofrequency ablation for treatment of pediatric atrioventricular nodal reentrant tachycardia: initial experience with 4-mm cryocatheter. Heart Rhythm. 2006;3:564–70.

27. Chanani NK, Chiesa NA, Dubin AM, et al. Cryoablation for atrioventricular nodal reentrant tachycardia in young patients: predictors of recurrence. Pacing Clin Electrophysiol. 2008;31:1152–9.

28. Bar-Cohen Y, Cecchin F, Alexander ME, et al. Cryoablation for accessory pathways located near normal conduction tissues or within the coronary venous system in children and young adults. Heart Rhythm. 2006;3:253–8.

29. Avari JN, Jay KS, Rhee EK. Experience and results during transition from radiofrequency ablation to cryoablation for treatment of pediatric atrioventricular nodal reentrant tachycardia. Pacing Clin Electrophysiol. 2008;31:454–60.

30. Saul JP, Hulse JE, Papagiannis J, et al. Late enlargement of radiofrequency lesions in infant lambs. Implications for ablation procedures in small children. Circulation. 1994;90:492–9.

31. Khairy P, Guerra PG, Rivard L, et al. Enlargement of catheter ablation lesions in infant hearts with cryothermal versus radiofrequency energy: an animal study. Circ Arrhythm Electrophysiol. 2011;4:211–7.

32. Kriebel T, Hermann HP, Schneider H, et al. Cryoablation at growing myocardium: no evidence of coronary artery obstruction or intimal plaque formation early and late after energy application. Pacing Clin Electrophysiol. 2009;32:1197–202.

33. Fischbach PS, Saarel EV, Dick M, 2nd. Transient atrioventricular conduction block with cryoablation following normal cryomapping. Heart Rhythm. 2004;1:554–7.

34. Drago F, Silvetti MS, De Santis A, et al. Lengthier cryoablation and a bonus cryoapplication is associated with improved efficacy for cryothermal catheter ablation of supraventricular tachycardias in children. J Interv Card Electrophysiol. 2006;16:191–8.

35. Miyazaki A, Blaufox AD, Fairbrother DL, et al. Prolongation of the fast pathway effective refractory period during cryoablation in children: a marker of slow pathway modification. Heart Rhythm. 2005;2:1179–85.

36. Kaltman JR, Tanel RE, Wegrzynowicz B, et al. Time and temperature profile of catheter cryoablation of right septal and free wall accessory pathways in children. J Cardiovasc Electrophysiol. 2008;19:343–7.

37. Drago F, Russo MS, Silvetti MS, et al. "Time to effect" during cryomapping: a parameter related to the long-term success of accessory pathways cryoablation in children. Europace. 2009;11:630–4.

38. Law IH, Von Bergen NH, Gingerich JC, et al. Transcatheter cryothermal ablation of junctional ectopic tachycardia in the normal heart. Heart Rhythm. 2006;3:903–7.

39. Von Bergen NH, Abu Rasheed H, Law IH. Transcatheter cryoablation with 3-D mapping of an atrial ectopic tachycardia in a pediatric patient with tachycardia induced heart failure. J Interv Card Electrophysiol. 2007;18:273–9.

40. McCanta AC, Kay JD, Collins KK. Cryoablation of the slow atrioventricular nodal pathway via a transbaffle approach in a patient with the Mustard procedure for D-transposition of the great arteries. Congenit Heart Dis. 2011;6:479–83.

41. Gist K, Tigges C, Smith G, et al. Learning curve for zero-fluoroscopy catheter ablation of AVNRT: early versus late experience. Pacing Clin Electrophysiol. 2011;34:264–8.

Atrioventricular Nodal Reentrant Tachycardia: What Have We Learned from Radiofrequency Catheter Ablation?

Ruey J. Sung,[1] Charlie Young,[2] and Michael R. Lauer[2]

[1]Stanford University School of Medicine, Stanford, CA, USA
[2]Kaiser-Permanente Medical Center, San Jose, CA, USA

Introduction

Atrioventricular (AV) nodal reentrant tachycardia (AVNRT) is the most common form of paroxysmal supraventricular tachycardia encountered in clinical practice.[1] Its prevalence is noted to increase in young adults after puberty, and there is a marked female preponderance. Characteristically, AVNRT has an abrupt onset and offset, and its termination can be facilitated by vagal maneuvers. Depending on the rate and duration of the tachycardia, clinical symptoms associated with the arrhythmia vary among individuals, including palpitations, lightheadedness, dyspnea, chest discomfort, and rarely syncope. Although most patients do not have structural heat disease, long-lasting and incessant tachycardia[2] may lead to development of tachycardia-induced cardiomyopathy.[3]

Since 1990, the technique of catheter ablation has evolved to become an effective modality for managing symptomatic patients with drug-refractory AVNRT.[4–8] In this presentation, we intend to review what we have learned from radiofrequency catheter ablation (RFCA) in the treatment of AVNRT over the past 20 years.

Basis of catheter ablation for AVNRT

The search for the electrophysiologic mechanism underpinning AVNRT dates back to the mid-1900s. In 1966, using microelectrode recording, Moe and Mendez[9] demonstrated that reciprocal rhythm (i.e., atrial and ventricular echoes) and intranodal circus movement could be induced by premature stimulation within the AV node in isolated rabbit hearts, substantiating their indirect observations previously made in the dog heart.[10] They postulated that the upper part of the AV node could undergo "functional dissociation" into two conducting pathways (α and β) differing in electrophysiologic properties, which converged distally to form a distal common pathway above the bundle of His.[9–11] Subsequently, utilizing a "brush electrode" containing 10 microelectrodes, Janse et al.[12–14] illustrated dual AV nodal inputs at the low crista terminalis and the low interatrial septum and confirmed the inducibility of AVNRT in isolated rabbit hearts. They further surmised that "functional longitudinal dissociation" of the AV node was the underlying mechanism of AVNRT.

In 1968, Schuilenburg et al.[15] applied the concept of "dual AV nodal physiology" to explain the occur-

The Practice of Catheter Cryoablation for Cardiac Arrhythmias, First Edition. Edited by Ngai-Yin Chan.
© 2014 John Wiley & Sons, Ltd. Published 2014 by John Wiley & Sons, Ltd.

rence of atrial echoes elicited by atrial premature beats in the human heart. In 1973, applying the technique of His bundle recording in humans,[16] Rosen et al.[17,18] showed that atrial premature stimulation could induce "dual AV nodal physiology," reflected as discontinuous AV nodal conduction (A_1–A_2;H_1–H_2) curves, and that the initiation of AVNRT was associated with such an electrophysiologic phenomenon. Accordingly, they supported the notion that "functional dissociation" of the AV node was the mechanism responsible for paroxysmal AVNRT in humans.

In 1981, inspired by these sequential research works, Sung et al.[19] performed intracardiac mapping using catheters with multiple electrodes in patients with "dual AV nodal physiology" and noted that the so-called slow AV nodal pathway (SP) had a sequence of retrograde atrial activation distinctly different from that of the fast AV nodal pathway (FP). Specifically, while the retrograde atrial exit of FP was very close to the His bundle recording site, that of SP was located posteriorly and inferiorly in the proximity of the coronary sinus (CS) ostium (Figure 3.1). They implied that "dual AV nodal physiology" was not only functional but also in actuality anatomical, and that the proximal common pathway was a broad area. These latter findings, later corroborated by Ross et al.[20] and McGuire et al.[21] in curative surgery and high-resolution mapping of the Koch's triangle in patients with AVNRT, respectively, have since become the cornerstone for selective catheter ablation of dual AV nodal pathway conduction for eliminating AVNRT in humans.[4–8]

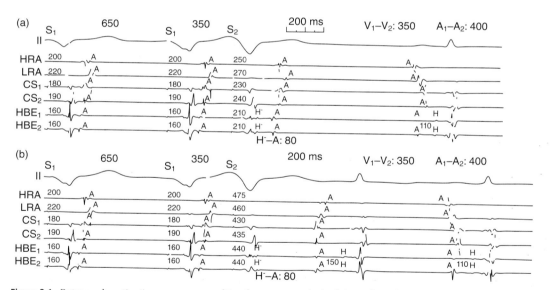

Figure 3.1. Retrograde activation sequence resulting from retrograde dual AV node pathway conduction. In each panel, from top to bottom, the surface electrocardiogram (ECG) lead II, along with intracardiac recordings from the high right atrium (HRA), lateral right atrium (LRA), coronary sinus ostium (CS_1), distal coronary sinus (CS_2), and proximal and distal His bundle regions (HBE_1 and HBE_2, respectively), are shown. The right ventricle is driven at a cycle length (S_1–S_1) of 650 ms. (a) A ventricular extrastimulus delivered with a premature coupling interval (S_1–S_2) of 350 ms produces ventriculo-atrial activation via retrograde FP (fast AV nodal pathway) conduction during which the earliest retrograde atrial exit is recorded at the HBE_1 region. (b) In the same patient, a ventricular extrastimulus delivered with the same premature coupling interval (S_1–S_2) of 350 ms can also produce ventriculo-atrial activation by way of retrograde SP (slow AV nodal pathway) conduction, during which, however, the earliest retrograde exit is registered at CS_1 (coronary sinus ostium).[19] (Source: Sung RJ, Wasman HL, Saksena S, Juma Z, 1981[19]. Reproduced with permission from Wolters Kluwer Health).

Techniques of radiofrequency catheter ablation

Following the introduction of radiofrequency (RF) current for catheter ablation,[22] the initial procedure targeted FP conduction via delivering RF current to the antero-superior aspect of the tricuspid annulus.[5–8] However, because of a high rate of producing complete AV block, selective ablation of SP conduction via delivering RF current to the postero-inferior septal right atrium close to the CS ostium[19] has become the method of choice.[5–8]

Electrophysiologic study

Selective ablation of SP conduction is applicable to all forms of AVNRT, that is, (typical) slow-fast, (atypical) fast-slow, and (variant) slow-slow,[5–7,23–25] which respectively constitute approximately 77%, 4.9%, and 11.6% of AVNRT patients undergoing electrophysiologic study (EPS) (with 6.5% undetermined).[25] In general, the ablation procedure is combined with a diagnostic EPS in a single session during which the mechanism of AVNRT and the coexistence of other arrhythmias such as atrial flutter, atrial tachycardia, ventricular tachycardia, and AV reciprocating tachycardia involving an accessory bypass tract[26] are either excluded or further identified for better therapeutic planning. For example, AVNRT has been found to not infrequently coexist with idiopathic ventricular tachycardia, which also has a high prevalence in young adults and is amenable to RFCA.[27,28] Moreover, fast-slow AVNRT may clinically present as an incessant tachycardia that needs to be differentiated from the permanent form of junctional reciprocating tachycardia, often referred to as PJRT, involving a decremental conducting bypass tract.[2] Under these circumstances, detailed mapping of the retrograde atrial activation sequence coupled with a stable recording of the His bundle potential during EPS is essential for defining the precise mechanism and for determining the proper site to which RF current should be delivered. The protocol of diagnostic EPS for AVNRT can be readily found in the literature.[23–29]

Briefly, the EPS protocol consists of programmed atrial and ventricular electrical stimulation at two cycle lengths (usually 600 and 400 ms, respectively) with extrastimulation and incremental pacing respectively performed in the atrium and the ventricle. Discontinuous AV nodal conduction $(A_1–A_2;H_1–H_2)$ curves are defined as the induction of 50 ms (40 ms for pediatric patients) or more A–H interval jumps in response to 10 ms decrements of the coupling interval of a single atrial extrastimulus.[17,18] In case AVNRT is not inducible at baseline, isoproterenol (0.5 to 3 μg/min) is infused, if there are no contraindications, to increase the sinus rate by 25%, and the protocol of programmed electrical stimulation is repeated.[29,30] Isoproterenol enhances conduction of the anterograde SP and/or retrograde FP, thereby facilitating induction of AVNRT.[29,30] At the completion of the ablation procedure, the inducibility of AVNRT as described in this chapter is tested in all patients.

Electrophysiologically, modes of initiation and termination of AVNRT with programmed electrical stimulation (i.e., extrastimulation and incremental pacing) are in accordance with the mechanism of reentry.[31–34] Besides, the presence of a wide excitable gap that can be demonstrated in both FP (antero-superior interatrial septum) and SP (postero-inferior interatrial septum) areas, occupying one-third ($34 \pm 9\%$ and $33 \pm 11\%$, respectively) of the tachycardia cycle length (significantly more than those of the high right atrium, proximal CS, and right ventricular apex [$3 \pm 9\%$, $24 \pm 11\%$, and $4 \pm 6\%$, respectively]),[35] is also consistent with the mechanism of reentry.[31–34] Furthermore, both FP and SP can have separate atrial inputs not only in the retrograde but also in the anterograde direction,[36] and an atrial extrastimulus delivered from either the FP or SP area can capture the respective atrial tissue and transmit the impulse through anterograde FP to reach the His bundle without interrupting the tachycardia (i.e., resetting of the tachycardia) (Figure 3.2).[35] Taken together, these electrophysiological findings imply that both FP and SP are distinctly different anatomical tissues involved in "dual AV nodal physiology" and the reentrant circuit of AVNRT.

Combined anatomical and electrophysiological approach

Different techniques for catheter ablation of SP conduction have been elaborated.[6–8] Bearing some variation among different medical centers, a combined

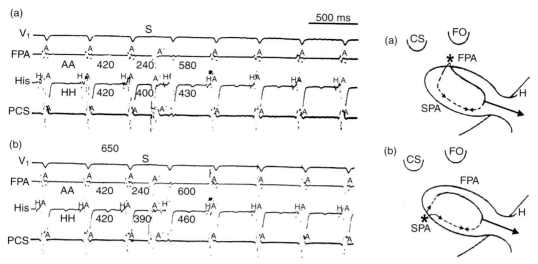

Figure 3.2. Resetting of slow-fast AVNRT with atrial extrastimulation within the excitable gap. A single atrial extrastimulus (S) with a premature coupling interval of 240 ms delivered from either the FP (fast AV nodal pathway; (a)) or SP (slow AV nodal pathway; (b)) area resets slow-fast atrioventricular nodal reentrant tachycardia (AVNRT) with a cycle length of 420 ms. Note that despite being in a slow-fast form (i.e., using SP for anterograde conduction and FP for retrograde conduction), the atrial extrastimulus (S) captures the respective atrium (A′) and transmits the impulse through anterograde FP to reach the His bundle (A′–H′), but allows the subsequent anterograde SP conduction to continue (reaching the His bundle, H″), sustaining the slow-fast form of AVNRT. These latter events are attested by an atrial extrastimulus-induced short A′–H′ interval followed by lengthening of the H′–H″ interval to 430 ms (a) and 450 ms (b) (control H–H interval during the tachycardia: 420 ms). This unique mechanism of resetting supports that both FP and SP are distinctly different anatomical tissues involved in the reentrant circuit of slow-fast AVNRT. PCS: proximal coronary sinus; His: His bundle electrographic lead. (Source: Lai WT, Lee CS, Sheu SH, Hwang YS, Sung RJ, 1995[35]. Reproduced with permission from Wolters Kluwer Health).

anatomical and electrophysiological approach is generally utilized. Before deployment of a steerable 7 French mapping and ablation catheter, three electrode catheters are placed in the high right atrium, right ventricular apex, and CS, respectively. For mapping and ablation purposes, a biplane fluoroscopy is available to all patients. The SP region[19] is targeted for catheter ablation in all patients. The tip (4 mm electrode) of the steerable mapping and ablation catheter is directed to the inferior region of the vestibule of the tricuspid valve below the CS ostium. Between the 4 mm electrode and an adhesive skin electrode in the right thigh, RF current is delivered via a power supply as a continuous, unmodulated sine wave output at 500 kHz (30–50 W). In patients in whom the earliest retrograde exit of SP is identifiable, as is usually the case with fast-slow AVNRT, RF current is applied directly to that site. Otherwise, in

most patients who exclusively exhibit retrograde FP conduction, mapping is performed via the ablation electrode pair along the tricuspid annulus from the CS ostium to the His bundle electrogram recording site (the Koch triangle),[5–8,19] which can be divided into three zones (A, anterior; M, middle; and P, posterior) (Figures 3.3 and 3.4). The electrogram obtained from the ablation electrode pair before delivery of RF current should exhibit an atrial-to-ventricular electrogram ratio of ≤0.25 (i.e., a large ventricular potential and a small atrial potential, with or without fractionated deflections – "slow pathway potentials"[37]). During ablation, a stable recording of the His bundle potential is ensured, and a brief period of bipolar pacing (4–6 beats) through the ablation electrode pair may be performed to ascertain capture of the target tissue. Delivery of RF current is systematically commenced posteriorly

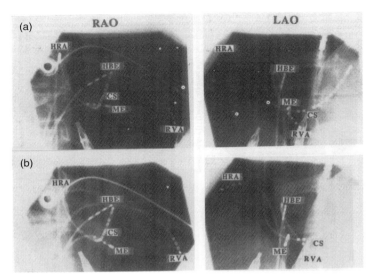

Figure 3.3. Fluoroscopic radiograph of the position of the catheter ablation mapping electrode (ME) taken from right anterior oblique (RAO) and left anterior oblique (LAO) views. (a) The 4 mm distal electrode (ME) is positioned in the posterior (P) region corresponding to the lower third of the Koch triangle – the His bundle electrogram (HBE)–coronary sinus (CS) ostium axis. This position is designated P_1 (i.e., the anterior half of the P region). (b) The ME is also positioned in the P region, but is located approximately 1 cm inferior and posterior to the CS ostium referred to as P_2 (i.e., the posterior half of the P region) (see text). HRA, high right atrium; RVA: right ventricular apex. (Source: Sung RJ, Lauer MR, 2000[63]. Copyright © 2000, Springer. With kind permission from Springer Science + Business Media B.V.).

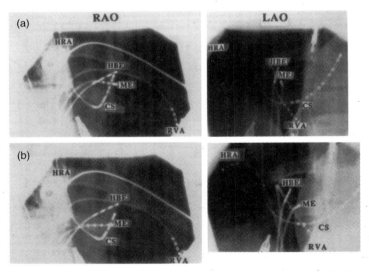

Figure 3.4. Fluoroscopic radiograph of the position of the catheter ablation mapping electrode (ME) taken from right anterior oblique (RAO) and left anterior oblique (LAO) views. (a) The 4 mm distal electrode (ME) is positioned in the anterior (A) region corresponding to the upper third of the Koch triangle – the His bundle electrogram (HBE)–coronary sinus (CS) ostium axis. (b) The ME is positioned in the middle (M) region, corresponding to the middle third of the Koch triangle. HRA, high right atrium; RVA: right ventricular apex. (Source: Sung RJ, Lauer MR, 2000[63]. Copyright © 2000, Springer. With kind permission from Springer Science + Business Media B.V.).

near the CS ostium (P zone) and proceeds anteriorly (M and A zones) (Figures 3.3 and 3.4). The RF energy delivery is to achieve an electrode–tissue interface temperature of approximately 55 °C for 30–60 seconds. In each attempt, application of RF energy is guided by the emergence of a junctional ectopic rhythm (five or more beats, regular or irregular).[38–40] The junctional ectopic rhythm so induced is temperature dependent, the mean appearance time of which is 8.8 ± 4.1 sec. For predicting successful ablation, the emergence of such a rhythm has a sensitivity of 98%, specificity of 57%, and negative predictive value of 99%.[39] Hence, no such rhythm appearing within 10–15 seconds after initiation of RF energy delivery should prompt termination of the RF application and repositioning of the ablation catheter. The application of RF energy is also immediately stopped if there is loss of 1-to-1 retrograde atrial activation noted during the junctional ectopic rhythm, or if there is visible prolongation of the AH interval during sinus rhythm or of the H–A interval during the junctional ectopic rhythm.[37–40] Additionally, if the rate of junction ectopic rhythm is fast (>100/min), the delivery of RF energy is discontinued immediately to avoid complete AV block. If the electrode–tissue interface temperature is less than 50 °C, multiple applications of RF energy are often required for successful ablation. Following a seemingly successful attempt, AV nodal conduction is reassessed using programmed electrical stimulation. Complete loss of "dual AV nodal physiology" (i.e., discontinuous A_1–A_2;H_1–H_2 curves) is not necessary for long-term symptomatic relief of the arrhythmia.[41–43] The most widely accepted endpoint for immediate success is noninducibility of the arrhythmia with or without isoproterenol infusion. In other words, inducible single echo beats (i.e., no more than one) with programmed atrial stimulation are considered acceptable endpoints and defined as "SP modification." Whether isoproterenol infusion should be routinely challenged post ablation is debatable. Intuitively speaking, it should be tested in those patients in whom isoproterenol infusion is required for the induction of AVNRT at baseline (Figure 3.5).[43,44]

Variation of retrograde exit sites and presence of multiple AV nodal pathways

The anatomy and cellular architecture of the AV junction, including the AV node proper and its surrounding tissues, in humans are complex.[46–49] Morphologic changes of the human AV node appear to be age dependent, which may account for the increase in the prevalence of AVNRT in young adults after puberty.[48] During catheter ablation, functional anterograde FP may at times be found at the posteroseptal right atrium where SP modification is usually performed (Figures 3.6 and 3.7),[50] and rarely, even in patients with a normal heart, the retrograde exit of either FP or SP can occasionally be registered at the left atrial septum.[51]

Furthermore, multiple AV nodal pathways with variable atrial insertion sites into the AV node may be present (Figure 3.8). Findings of EPS[25,41–54] are in line with the notion that the anatomic correlate for multiple slow pathways could be rightward and leftward inferior extensions of the AV node.[46–49] Of interest, Sinkovec et al.[52] performed atrial extrastimulation from the right atrial appendage and the posterolateral CS to test right atrial and left atrial inputs, respectively, in 29 patients with slow-fast AVNRT under pharmacological autonomic blockade. They could demonstrate discordance of conduction velocity, refractoriness, and parasympathetic modulation between right and left atrial inputs. Relevant to catheter ablation of AVNRT, Lee et al.[53] noted that 7 (9%) of 78 patients with AVNRT undergoing EPS exhibited two discrete discontinuities in AV nodal conduction (A_1–A_2;H_1–H_2) curves, suggestive of the presence of triple (fast, intermediate, and slow) AV nodal pathways. Detailed mapping of the retrograde atrial activation sequence showed that the retrograde exit site of these three pathways varied somewhat in the three zones (A, M, and P) (Figure 3.8): the FP was anterior (4/7) and middle (3/7), the intermediate pathway was middle (4/7) and posterior (3/7), and the SP was middle (1/7) and posterior (6/7). Functionally, they could also show (1) triple ventricular depolarizations resulting from a single atrial impulse, (2) sequential dual ventricular echoes, (3) spontaneous transformation between slow-fast and fast-slow forms of AVNRT, and (4) cycle length alternans during AVNRT. Additionally, they illustrated that all three pathways could be involved in AV nodal echoes or AVNRT. Therefore, the reentrant circuit of AVNRT in the fast-slow form may or may not be exactly the reverse of the slow-fast form.[25] All the findings given here emphasize the importance of detailed mapping and localization of

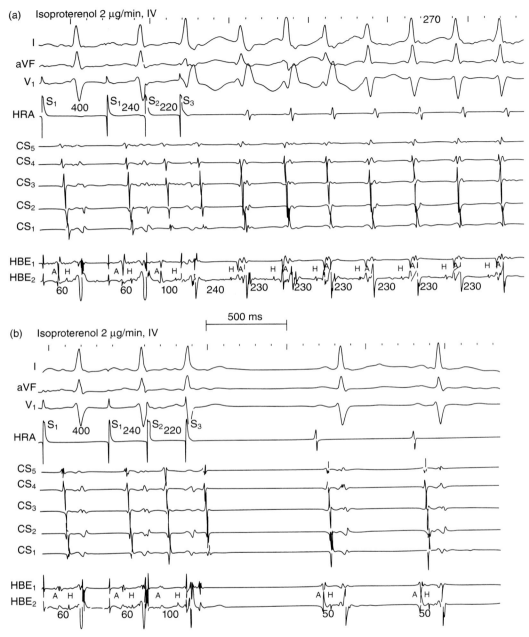

Figure 3.5. Selective ablation of slow atrioventricular (AV) nodal pathway (SP) conduction. From top to bottom in each panel, surface electrocardiogram (ECG) leads II, aVF, and V_1, along with intracardiac recordings from the high right atrium (HRA), proximal and distal coronary sinus (CS_1 and CS_2, respectively), and proximal and distal His bundle regions (HBE_1 and HBE_2, respectively), are shown. (a) At baseline, isoproterenol infusion at 2 μg/min coupled with two atrial extrastimuli (S_2 and S_3) are required to expose anterograde SP conduction (A–H interval: 240 ms) for induction of slow-fast AV nodal reentrant tachycardia (AVNRT) (cycle length: 270 ms) during HRA pacing (S_1–S1 = 400 ms). (b) Application of RF energy to site P_1 close to CS_1 (coronary sinus ostium) successfully abolishes anterograde SP conduction and renders the tachycardia noninducible even under isoproterenol challenge coupled with two atrial extrastimuli (S_2 and S_3). A: atrial electrogram; H: His bundle potential; CS_1–CS_5: distal to proximal coronary sinus. (Source: Huycke EC, Lai WT, Nguyen NX, Keung EC, Sung RJ, 1989[29]. Reproduced with permission from Elsevier, Copyright © 1989 Elsevier).

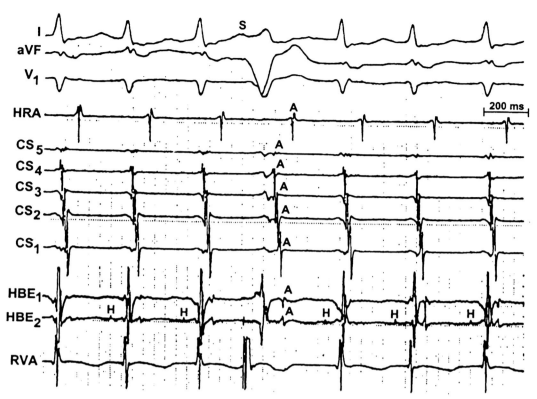

Figure 3.6. Unusual retrograde atrial activation sequence resulting from retrograde fast AV nodal pathway (FP) conduction. An extrastimulus (S) is delivered at the right ventricular apex (RVA) during slow-fast atrioventricular nodal reentrant tachycardia (AVNRT) (VA interval <90 ms). The resultant premature ventricular capture separates the atrial electrogram from the ventricular electrogram, thereby allowing better analysis of the retrograde atrial activation sequence during the tachycardia. Note that the atrial electrogram recorded from the coronary sinus ostium (CS$_5$) precedes low septal right atrial (HBE$_1$ and HBE$_2$) and high right atrial (HRA) activation. In this situation, differential diagnosis should include slow-intermediate and slow-slow AVNRT. A: atrial electrogram; H: His bundle potential; CS$_1$–CS$_5$: distal to proximal coronary sinus. (Source: Sung RJ, Lauer MR, 2000[63]. Copyright © 2000, Springer. With kind permission from Springer Science + Business Media B.V.).

the retrograde atrial exit site of both FP and SP, whenever possible, before RF energy application in attempting catheter ablation of AVNRT (Figures 3.6 and 3.7).

Congenital heart disease

The AV node and the surrounding tissues are often anatomically distorted, and the course of the AV fibers into the SP is not uncommonly altered in patients with congenital heart disease.[55–62] For example, in patients with endocardial cushion defects, the AV node–His bundle system is usually displaced posteriorly and inferiorly at the AV junction.[55] Even in patients with atrial septal defects, the His bundle can be located at the CS ostium with reversal of FP and SP inputs into the AV node.[56] Likewise, in some patients, the CS ostium can be directly connected to the left atrium, and the AV node–His bundle system is located in the left atrium; selective ablation of SP conduction can be accomplished only by delivery of RF energy in the left atrial septal region.[59,62]

Under these circumstances, it is difficult to apply standard anatomic landmarks for locating FP and

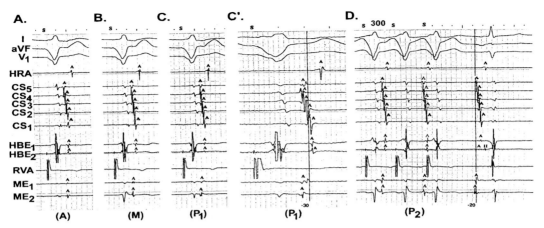

Figure 3.7. Mapping of earliest retrograde atrial exit sites of fast and slow AV nodal pathways (FP and SP, respectively) in the same patient as in Figure 3.6. The atrial electrogram recorded from the distal mapping electrode (ME$_2$) of the ablation catheter relative to those recorded from the coronary sinus ostium (CS$_5$), low right atrial septum (HBE$_1$ and HBE$_2$), and high right atrium (HRA) in the A, M, P$_1$, and P$_2$ regions during right ventricular apical (RVA) pacing (S) is displayed at the bottom trace of each panel. Paper speed is 100 mm/sec in panels A, B, C, and D, and 250 mm/sec in panel C′. Note that the earliest retrograde atrial exit site resulting from retrograde FP conduction recorded at ME$_2$ is in the P$_1$ region, which is −30 ms from the onset of atrial electrogram registered at HBE$_1$ (denoted by a vertical line in panel C′). In panel D, the RVA pacing cycle length (S–S) is shortened from 400 ms to 300 ms. Note that the third ventricular-paced beat induces a ventricular (AV node) echo that is preceded by a marked prolongation of ventriculo-atrial conduction time due to sifting of retrograde FP (the first and second ventricular-paced beats) to retrograde SP conduction accompanied by a change in the retrograde atrial activation sequence. The earliest retrograde atrial exit site resulting from retrograde SP conduction is recorded in the P$_2$ region, which is −20 ms from the onset of the atrial electrogram registered at CS$_5$ (the coronary sinus ostium) (denoted by a vertical line in panel D). Hence, in this case, earliest retrograde atrial exits of FP and SP are located very close to each other (i.e., P$_1$ and P$_2$, respectively). This atrioventricular nodal reentrant tachycardia may be interpreted as an intermediate-slow form, with retrograde FP being an "intermediate" AV nodal pathway. A: atrial electrogram; H: His bundle potential; CS$_1$-CS$_5$: distal to proximal coronary sinus. (Source: Sung RJ, Lauer MR, 2000[63]. Copyright © 2000, Springer. With kind permission from Springer Science + Business Media B.V.).

SP areas, and the potential risk of inadvertent AV block is increased. Nevertheless, with the aid of right atriogram and biplane fluoroscopy for defining the anatomical structure and for recording the His bundle potential, successful catheter ablation of AVNRT has been reported in patients with various congenital heart diseases, such as atresia of the CS ostium, complete situs inversus, persistent left superior vena cava, repaired incomplete endocardial cushion defects, and so on.[57–62]

Potential proarrhythmic effects of catheter ablation

During the process of selective ablation of either FP or SP conduction, proarrhythmic effects may be observed during the initial application of RF current. Since "slow conduction" is one of the prerequisites favoring reentry,[31–34] proarrhythmic effects are expected to occur more often with selective FP than with selective SP ablation (Table 3.1).[63] Specifically, while attempting selective FP ablation, (1) elimination of anterograde FP conduction alone can enhance the inducibilty of typical slow-fast AVNRT; (2) elimination of retrograde FP conduction alone may lead to atypical fast-slow AVNRT via unmasking retrograde SP conduction (Figure 3.9), which clinically often manifests as an incessant form of AVNRT[2] (in either case, repeated attempts to ablate the residual retrograde or anterograde FP conduction, respectively, would increase the risk of high-degree or complete AV block);[64] and (3) elimination of FP conduction in both anterograde and retrograde directions may unveil clinically silent AV reciprocating tachycardia using anterograde SP for

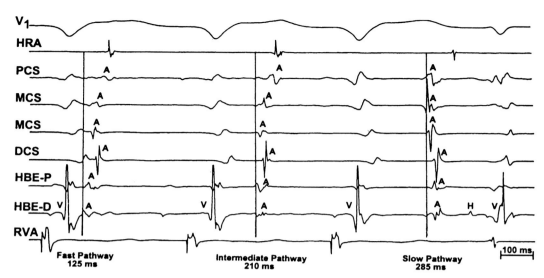

Figure 3.8. Three discrete retrograde atrioventricular (AV) nodal conduction pathways unveiled by ventricular pacing. Surface electrocardiogram (ECG) lead V_1 and intracardiac recordings of the high right atrium (HRA); proximal, middle, and distal coronary sinus (PCS, MCS, and DCS, respectively); proximal and distal His bundle regions (HBE-P and HBE-D, respectively); and right ventricular apical (RVA) electrograms are displayed. During RVA pacing at a cycle length of 450 ms, three different sequences of retrograde atrial activation can be identified. Based on differences in ventriculo-atrial conduction time as listed at the bottom of the figure in milliseconds (ms), the earliest retrograde exit of fast pathway (FP) is registered at the HBE-D recording site, that of the intermediate pathway at MCS, and that of the slow pathway (SP) at PCS near the coronary sinus ostium. The last QRS complex is a ventricular (AV node) echo produced by retrograde SP conduction followed by anterograde FP conduction. (Source: Lee KJ, Chun HM, Liem B, Lauer MR, Young C, Sung RJ, 1998[53]. Reproduced with permission from John Wiley and Sons Ltd).

Table 3.1. Potential proarrhythmic effects of RF catheter ablation at the AV junction

Conduction pathway	Anterograde	Retrograde	Proarrhythmic mechanism
Fast	+	−	Slow-fast atrioventricular nodal reentrant tachycardia (AVNRT)
Fast	−	+	Fast-slow AVNRT
Fast	+	+	Slow-AP RT*
Slow	+	−	Unlikely
Slow	−	+	Unlikely
Slow	+	+	Unlikely

*Slow-AP RT: Atrioventricular reciprocating tachycardia using a slow pathway (SP) for anterograde conduction and a concealed bypass tract (AP) for retrograde conduction; +: ablation successful; −: ablation unsuccessful.

anterograde conduction and a concealed AV bypass tract for retrograde conduction. Notably, Silka et al.[64] reported that the incidence of transforming typical slow-fast to atypical fast-slow AVNRT during RFCA could be as high as 28% (5 of 18) in children (mean age: 12.9 ± 3.4 years) compared to only 3.4% (2 of 59) in adult patients ($p = 0.01$). They ascribed the high incidence of this proarrhythmic effect to the difference in the anatomic and electro-physiologic substrates of the AV junction that evolve as a function of age.[48]

In contrast, while attempting selective SP ablation, elimination of anterograde SP conduction alone or of both anterograde and retrograde SP conductions

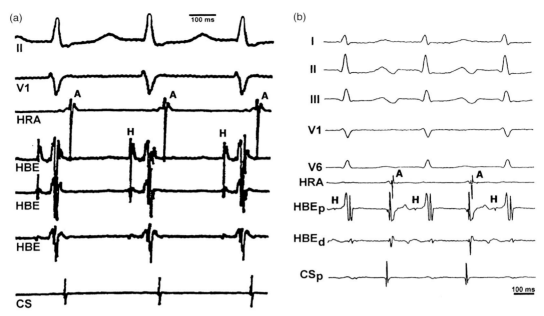

Figure 3.9. Facilitation of induction of fast-slow atrioventricular nodal reentrant tachycardia (AVNRT) after ablation-induced abolition of retrograde fast pathway (FP) conduction. (a) Slow-fast AVNRT induced at baseline. (b) After an attempt of radiofrequency catheter ablation that has resulted in elimination of retrograde FP conduction alone, fast-slow AVNRT becomes readily inducible due to unmasking of retrograde slow pathway (SP) conduction. CS, coronary sinus; d: distal; HBE: His bundle electrographic lead; HRA: high right atrium; p: proximal. (Source: Sung RJ, Lauer MR, 2000[63]. Copyright © 2000, Springer. With kind permission from Springer Science + Business Media B.V.).

is unlikely to be proarrhythmic because of the presence of retrograde FP conduction. However, elimination of SP in the retrograde direction alone or in both anterograde and retrograde directions admittedly may uncover the presence of other SPs,[65] triggering onset of (variant) slow-slow AVNRT.[63]

Safety and efficacy of RFCA

Immediate results
Selective ablation of either FP or SP conduction is an effective means for eliminating AV nodal reentry.[4–8] However, selective FP ablation is associated with a high rate of inadvertent AV block. Jazayeri et al.[5] performed selective FP ablation in a series of 19 patients, including 3 who had previously failed selective SP ablation. Despite successful abolition of the arrhythmia inducibility in all (100%), four of them (22%) developed complete AV block. They also attempted selective SP ablation in another series of 33 patients. Complete abolition of the arrhythmia inducibility was accomplished

in 32 of them (97%), and all of them maintained intact AV conduction. In a series of 80 patients undergoing selective SP ablation, Jackman et al.[6] reported a success rate of 100% (80 of 80) and 1.3% (1 of 80) of inadvertent AV block. These two groups of investigators[4,6] as well as others[7,8] concluded that selective ablation of SP conduction was a safe and effective means of eliminating AV nodal reentry and should be considered the procedure of choice in managing patients with recurrent AVNRT. After progression through a learning curve for the procedural skills conjoined with advances in the ablation technology, the success rate of selective SP ablation for the treatment of AVNRT is estimated to be 95%, and the risk of complete AV block requiring permanent pacemaker therapy <1% (0.5–3.0%).[66–72]

Short- and long-term follow-up evaluation
The recurrence rate of the arrhythmia following the ablation procedure is relatively low, averaging <10% (0–13%).[66–72]

Of major concern is the long-term outcome of patients who have inadvertently induced transient AV block during the ablation procedure. In 186 consecutive AVNRT patients, Fenelon et al.[73] observed that late complete AV block occurred in 5 (26%) of the 19 patients who had had transient AV block (mean 2.8 ± 7.0 min), but none in those (167 patients) without this complication ($p = 0.0001$) during follow-up evaluation for 8.6 ± 8.3 and 10.1 ± 9.4 months, respectively. Of note, four of these five patients had FP ablation and the one who had SP ablation manifested asymptomatic 2 : 1 AV block during exercise. Kimman et al.[74] made a 10-year follow-up evaluation in 120 patients who underwent RFCA for AVNRT between 1991 and 1995, and noted that all of them were free from AVNRT recurrence, but 29 patients (24%) suffered from new arrhythmias such as atrial flutter (6), atrial tachycardia (6), atrial fibrillation (9), premature atrial contractions (16), and late AV block (2). They concluded that RF energy was potentially proarrhythmic and advocated the need to search for alternative energy sources. Similarly, in a cohort of 109 consecutive AVNRT patients who had undergone SP ablation, Arimoto et al.[75] noted no occurrence of late AV block during a mean follow-up period of 60.6 months despite the fact that the elderly (>55 years old) tended to have a significantly greater change in the PR interval from before ablation compared with the younger counterpart (<55 years old). Of note, they observed that older patients were more likely to develop atrial fibrillation (5 of 54 [9.3%]) compared with the younger group (0 of 44 [0%]), which could be attributed to the age-related presence of atrial vulnerability (positive inducibility of atrial fibrillation during EPS).

Elderly population

Several investigators have addressed the issue of safety and efficacy of RFCA of AVNRT in the elderly.[45,71,76-82] Kalusche et al.[76] analyzed results of RFCA for recurrent AVNRT in a series of 395 patients with a mean age of 52.3 (19–90) years. They noted that elderly patients ($n = 85$, mean age 70.4 years) more often had structural heart disease (e.g., atherosclerotic heart disease) (19.3% vs. 2.6%; $P < 0.02$), syncope or presyncope caused by the arrhythmia (43.2% vs. 29.8%; $P < 0.05$), and more hospitalizations and emergency treatments due to arrhythmia-related symptomatology (56.8% vs. 39.5%; $P < 0.05$) despite their inducible AVNRT having a slower rate compared to the younger subgroup (cycle length, 368 vs. 325 ms; $P < 0.001$). Of the total cohort, most underwent selective SP ablation (82% of the elderly vs. 94% of the young). The overall success rate was similar in both subgroups (95.3% vs. 96.8%), as was the recurrence rate (5.8% vs. 4.9%). Moreover, there were no differences in the fluoroscopy time, radiation exposure, and incidence of high-degree AV block (2.3% vs. 1.6%). Thus, in view that AVNRT might lead to severe and even life-threatening symptoms, they recommended that RFCA be considered as the first-choice therapeutic modality in the elderly. Rostock et al.[45] noted that patients who were 75 years or older ($n = 70$) were more likely to have a preexisting prolonged PR interval compared to those younger than 75 years ($n = 508$) (37% vs. 3.3%). However, surprisingly, development of AV block (0.79%) and recurrence of AVNRT (2.95%) were observed in the younger subgroup, but not in the older subgroup, after successful SP ablation with a follow-up period of 37 months. In a total number of 350 patients, Meiltz and Zimmermann[78] found that the elderly cohort (age $\geq$ 65 years; $n = 70$) more often had structural heart disease and age-related alteration of atrial-His (AH) and His-ventricular (HV) intervals compared to the younger group (age < 65 years; $n = 280$). The success rate of selective SP ablation was similar in both groups (70/70 vs. 277/280, $P = 0.38$), but inadvertent complete AV block (0 of 70 [0%] vs. 2 of 280 [0.57%]) and arrhythmia recurrence (0 of 70 [0%] vs. 16 of 280 [5.7%], $P = 0.001$) were seen only in the patients from the younger subgroup.

Although selective SP ablation can be safely performed in the elderly, special caution should be taken when ablation is targeted at the SP area in those with impaired AV conduction manifested as PR interval prolongation ($\geq$200 ms)[71,81-84] as development of both immediate and delayed high-degree AV block has been reported.[82,83] In a series of 18 patients with a mean age of 62 ± 7 years, Li et al.[82] reported that the incidence of delayed AV block following successful SP ablation was higher in patients with, compared to patients without, prolonged PR interval at baseline (6 of 18 vs. 0 of 328, $P < 0.001$). Of 33 elderly patients undergoing selective SP ablation, Reithmann et al.[83] described 3% (1 of 33) immediate and 10% (4 of 33) late AV block and, in addition, 9% (3 of 33, aged 66, 75, and 76 years) late sudden death of unknown causes during the follow-up (at 4, 16, and 48 months, respectively).

Most recently, in a cohort of 3234 patients from a German ablation registry who underwent catheter ablation (RF 97.7% and cryoablation 2.3%) of AVNRT, Hoffmann et al.[71] divided the cohort into three age groups: <50 years (group 1, $n = 1268$ [39.2%]; median age = 40 [30.0–45.0] years, 74.1% women), 50–75 years old (group 2, $n = 1707$ [52.8%]; 63.0 [58.0–69.0] years, 63.0% women), and >75 years old (group 3, $n = 259$ [8.0%]; 79.0 [77.0–82.0] years, 50.6% women). Procedure-related pericardial effusion occurred in five (0.3%) of group 2 and two (0.8%) of group 3 but in none of the group 1 ($P < 0.05$) patients. No differences were observed among the three groups with regard to success rate of catheter ablation (98.7% vs. 98.8% vs. 98.5%; $P = .92$) and the overall procedure duration (75.0 minutes [50.0–105.0]; $P = .93$). Complete AV block occurred in two of group 1 (0.2%) and six (0.4%) of group 2 but none of the group 3 patients ($P = 0.41$). During a median follow-up period of 1.4 years, AVNRT recurred in 5.7% of all patients. Compared with group 1 (2.0 days) or group 2 (2.0 days) patients, those >75 years old (group 3) had a significantly longer hospital stay (3.0 days) ($P < .0001$). Hoffmann et al.[71] concluded that, despite having a higher prevalence of structural heart disease, RFCA of AVNRT was a highly effective and safe procedure in the elderly. Moreover, due to the fact that the elderly are often intolerant of antiarrhythmic drug therapy, they suggested that RFCA should be considered the preferred treatment for AVNRT in this clinical setting.

Pediatric population

In a multicenter RFCA registry of 314 children and adolescents with AVNRT, Schaffer et al.[85] reported that the success rate was 90% and the incidence of inadvertent AV block was 1.6% (5 of 314), of which 5.9% (1 of 17) was associated with selective FP ablation and 1.3% (4 of 297) with selective SP ablation. However, in the Pediatric Radiofrequency Ablation Registry, Kugler et al.[86,87] described that the complication rate for AVNRT ablation appeared to be age dependent, and, of note, only 71% of the patients were free from arrhythmia recurrence at 3 years follow-up. Another important issue of concern is fluoroscopy time and radiation exposure

in this subset of patients. From data gathered between two eras (1991–1995 and 1996–1999), Kugler et al.[88] further showed that there was a significant improvement in RFCA for all types of arrhythmia in children. More specifically, overall the failure rate was decreased by 50%, mean fluoroscopy time decreased by 21%, along with a significant decrease in the rate of complication;[88] the average fluoroscopy time for RFCA of AVNRT registered a median of 16 min (range 7–33 min), which was comparable to that reported in the Pediatric Radiofrequency Ablation Registry.

Lessons learned from RFCA

Observations and experiences described in the literature have provided paramount information regarding the mechanism of AV nodal reentry, and precautious measures needed to be taken for therapeutic intervention in various clinical settings:

1. Although functional factors such as nonuniform anisotropy[49] cannot be completely ruled out, the presence of an anatomic basis responsible for AVNRT in humans is incontrovertible. That AVNRT generally involves two distinct areas, FP (antero-superior) and SP (postero-inferior), is evidenced by abolition of the arrhythmia inducibility following application of RF current to these two distinct areas, respectively. However, the location of reentrant circuits (i.e., slow-fast, fast-slow, and slow-slow) remains elusive as they have never been clearly demonstrated either anatomically or electrophysiologically.

2. While attempting selective ablation of SP conduction using RF energy, the emergence of an AV junctional rhythm often heralds successful modification of AV nodal reentry with a negative predictive value of 99%.[41] Notably, this AV junctional rhythm does not seem to originate from the endocardial site with which the ablation catheter tip has a close contact. Instead, it appears to exit remotely from the SP area (approximately 1.0 to 1.5 cm from the compact node), registering a retrograde atrial activation sequence similar to that of retrograde FP conduction (an antero-superior exit site).[37] Moreover, this rhythm does not occur when RF energy is delivered to the atrial tissue normally devoid of pacemaker activity (diastolic depolarization).[89] These findings are in accord with those illustrated by Thibault et al.[90] in isolated pig and rabbit hearts, in which heat–RF application in the area located over (or very close to) the compact AV node could induce two types of AV junctional automatic rhythm, one regular and the other irregular, the latter of which was presumably caused by interaction of multiple foci with conduction block occurring in the intervening tissues. Therefore, the SP area seems to be well connected to the AV node proper with tissues in between that can preferentially transmit the thermal effect of RF energy to the FP conduction area in the AV node.[39]

3. The dimension of the Koch triangle and structure of its neighboring tissues, including the CS, may vary considerably among individuals.[91,92] Potentially at higher risk of inadvertent AV block are patients with (a) unusual location of the earliest retrograde atrial exit site of either FP or SP (Figures 3.7 and 3.8); (b) a narrow dimension of the Koch triangle in which the earliest retrograde atrial exit sites of both FP and SP are located in proximity; and (c) preexisting AV conduction disturbance such as PR interval prolongation.[92,93]

Furthermore, clinically three subset groups of patients are expected to be at higher risk of inadvertent AV block: (a) elderly patients, especially those aged >75 years; (b) pediatric patients, in particular those aged <5 years, especially infants; and (c) those with congenital heart disease. The elderly often have significant structural heart disease and comorbid conditions affecting the lungs, liver, and kidneys. Besides technical difficulty, they are prone to complications, such as excessive bleeding, pneumothorax, pericardial effusion, pulmonary embolism, and so on. In children, and young adults as well, special concerns are fluoroscopy time and radiation exposure, and the need of lifelong pacemaker therapy in case of inadvertent AV block. In patients with congenital heart disease, the anatomy of the AV node–His-Purkinje system relative to the structure of the triangle of Koch is not uncommonly distorted. Consequently, the risk of inadvertent AV block is markedly increased.

4. Lastly, the RF current may not be the optimal energy source as RF-induced thermal injury causes tissue disruption with carbonization of the targeted tissue that increases the risk for perforation and thromboembolism. Indeed, there are needs to search for (a) an alternative energy to minimize inadvertent and late AV block (e.g., cryothermy guided by ice mapping seems as effective as but safer

than RFCA for curing AVNRT),[93] (b) a more accurate mapping system to better delineate the location of the triangle of Koch relative to the location of the His bundle and the CS ostium; and (c) more advanced technology to enable physicians to perform zero-fluoroscopic ablation procedures (e.g., intracardiac echocardiography, a nonfluoroscopic electroanatomical and electromagnetic mapping system).[94–96]

Conclusion

The evolution of our conceptual understanding of "dual AV nodal physiology" and the development of RFCA of SP conduction are exemplars of how medical advances can be made possible through concerted research endeavors of anatomists, surgeons, and basic and clinical electrophysiologists over a span of more than 5 decades. Today, RFCA of SP conduction as a procedure of curing AVNRT is accompanied by a high success rate, a low recurrence rate, and a low complication rate. Nevertheless, there are still shortcomings that need to be resolved. Of major concerns are the risk of inadvertent AV block and radiation exposure associated with prolonged fluoroscopic time, especially for children, young adults, and those with congenital heart disease. Further refinement of the technique and advancement of the technology remains necessary.

Acknowledgements

This work was in part supported by a grant from the Ministry of Education (Development Plan for World Class Universities and Research Centers of Excellence, National Central University), Taiwan.

References

1. Sung RJ, Lauer MR, Chun H. Atrioventricular nodal reentry current concepts and new perspectives. Pacing Clin Electrophysiol. 1994;17:1413–30.
2. Sung RJ. Incessant supraventricular tachycardia. Pacing Clin Electrophysiol. 1983;6:1306–26.
3. Furushima H, Chirnushi M, Sugiura H, et al. Radiofrequency catheter ablation for incessant atrioventricular nodal reentrant tachycardia normalized H-V block associated with tachycardia-induced cardiomyopathy J Electrocardiol. 2004;37:315–19.

4. Haissaguerre M, Warin JF, D'Ivernois C, *et al*. Fulguration for AV nodal tachycardia: results in 42 patients with a mean follow-up of 23 months. Pacing Clin Electrophysiol. 1990;13:2000–7.

5. Jazayeri Mr, Hempe SL, Sra JS, *et al*. Selective transcatheter ablation of the fast and slow pathways using radiofrequency energy in patients with atrioventricular nodal reentrant tachycardia. Circulation. 1992;85:1318–28.

6. Jackman WM, Beckman KJ, McCleland JH, *et al*. Treatment of supraventricular tachycardia due to atrioventricular nodal reentry by radiofrequency catheter ablation to slow pathway conduction. N Engl J Med. 1992;327:313–28.

7. Mitrani RD, Klein LS, Hackett FK, *et al*. Radiofrequency ablation for atrioventricular node reentrant tachycardia: comparison between fast (anterior) and slow (posterior) pathway ablation. J Am Coll Cardiol. 1993;21:432–41.

8. Kottkamp H, Hindricks G, Borggrefe M, *et al*. Radiofrequency catheter ablation of the anterosuperior and posteroinferior atrial approaches to the AV node for treatment of AV nodal reentrant tachycardia: techniques for selective ablation of "fast" and "slow" AV node pathways. J Cardiovasc Electrophysiol. 1997;8: 451–68.

9. Mendez C, Moe GK. Demonstration of a dual A-V nodal conduction system in the isolated rabbit heart. Circ Res. 1966;19:378–93.

10. Moe GK, Preston JB, Burlington H. Physiologic evidence of a dual AV transmission system. Circ Res. 1956;4:357–75.

11. Moe GK, Mendez C. The physiologic basis of reciprocal rhythm. Prog Cardiovasc Dis. 1966;8:461–82.

12. Janse MJ. Influence of the direction of the atrial wave front of A-V nodal transmission in isolated hearts of rabbits. Circ Res. 1969;25:439–49.

13. Janse MJ, Van Capelle FJ, Freud GE, *et al*. Circus movement within the AV node as a basis for supraventricular tachycardia as shown by multiple microelectrode recording in the Isolated rabbit heart. Circ Res. 1971; 28:403–14.

14. Van Capelle FJL, Janse MJ, Varghese PJ, *et al*. Spread of excitation in the atrioventricular node of isolated rabbit hearts studied by multiple microelectrode recording. Circ Res. 1972;31:602–16.

15. Schuilenburg RM, Durrer D. Atrial echo beats in the human heart elicited by induced atrial premature beats. Circulation. 1968;37:680–93.

16. Scherlag BJ, Lau SH, Helfant RH, *et al*. Catheter technique for recording His bundle activity in man. Circulation. 1969;39:13.

17. Rosen KM, Mehta A, Miller RA. Demonstration of dual atrioventricular nodal pathways in man. Am J Cardiol. 1974;33:291–4.

18. Denes P, Wu D, Dhingra RC, *et al*. Demonstration of dual A-V nodal pathways in patients with paroxysmal supraventricular tachycardia. Circulation. 1973;48: 549–55.

19. Sung RJ, Waxman HL, Saksena S, *et al*. Sequence of retrograde atrial activation in patients with dual atrioventricular nodal pathways. Circulation. 1981;64: 1059–67.

20. Ross DL, Jhonson DC, Dnniss AR, *et al*. Curative surgery for atrioventricular junctional ("AV nodal") reentrant tachycardia. J Am Coll Cardiol. 1985;6: 1383–92.

21. McGuire MA, Bourke JP, Robotin MC, *et al*. High resolution mapping of Koch's triangle using sixty electrodes in humans with atrioventricular junctional (AV nodal) reentrant tachycardia. Circulation. 1993; 88:2315–28.

22. Huang SK, Bharati S, Graham AR, *et al*. Closed-chest catheter desiccation of the atrioventricular junction using radiofrequency energy: A new method of catheter ablation. J Am Coll Cardiol. 1987;9:349–58.

23. Wu D, Denes P, Amat-y-Leon F, *et al*. An unusual variety of atrioventricular nodal reentry due to retrograde dual atrioventricular nodal pathways. Circulation. 1977;56:50.

24. Sung RJ, Styperek JL, Myerburg RJ, *et al*. Initiation of two distinct forms of atrioventricular nodal reentrant tachycardia during programmed ventricular stimulation in man. Am J Cardiol. 1978;42:404–15.

25. Heidbüchel H, Jackman WM. Characterization of subforms of AV nodal reentrant tachycardia. Europace. 2004;6:316–29.

26. Sung RJ, Styperek JL. Electrophysiologic identification of dual atrioventricular nodal pathway conduction in patients with accessory bypass tracts. Circulation. 1979;60:1464–76.

27. Kautzner J, Cihak R, Vancura V, *et al*. Coincidence of idiopathic ventricular outflow tract tachycardia and atrioventricular nodal reentrant tachycardia. Europace. 2003;5:215–20.

28. Kazemi B, Arya A, Haghjoo M, *et al*. Coincident atrioventricular nodal reentrant and idiopathic ventricular tachycardia. Asian Cardiovasc Thorac Ann. 2006; 14:284–8.

29. Huycke EC, Lai WT, Nguyen NX, *et al*. Role of intravenous isoproterenol in the electrophysiologic induction of atrioventricular node reentrant tachycardia in patients with dual atrioventricular node pathways. Am J Cardiol. 1989;64:1131–7.

30. Stellbrink C, Diem B, Schauerte P, *et al*. Differential effects of atropine and isoproterenol on inducibility of atrioventricular nodal reentrant tachycardia. J Interv Cardiol. 2001;5:463–9.

31. Mines GR. On dynamic equilibrium in the heart. J Physiol (London). 1913;46:349–83.

32. Lewis T. Observations upon flutter and fibrillation: IV. Impure flutter: theory of circus movement heart. Heart. 1920;7:293.

33. Moe GK, Pastelin G, Mendez R. Circus movement excitation of the atria. In Little RC, editor. Physiology of atrial pacemaker and conductive tissue. Mt. Kisco, NY: Futura Publishing; 1980. p. 207–20.

34. Allessie MA, Bonke FI, Schopman FJ. Circus movement in rabbit atrial muscle as a mechanism of tachycardia. Circ Res. 1973;33:54–62.

35. Lai WT, Lee CS, Sheu SH, et al. Electrophysiological manifestations of the excitable gap of slow-fast AV nodal reentrant tachycardia demonstrated by single extrastimulation. Circulation. 1995;92: 66–76.

36. Young C, Lauer MR, Liem LB, et al. Demonstration of a posterior atrial input to the atrioventricular node during sustained anterograde slow pathway conduction. J Am Coll Cardiol. 1998;31:1615–21.

37. Kuo CT, Lauer MR, Young C, et al. Electrophysiologic significance of discrete slow potential in patients with dual AV node physiology: implications for selection radiofrequency ablation of slow pathway conduction. Am Heart J. 1996;131:490–8.

38. Jentzer JH, Goyal R, Williamson BD, et al. Analysis of junctional ectopy during radiofrequency ablation of the slow pathway in patients with atrioventricular nodal reentrant tachycardia. Circulation. 1994;90: 2820–6.

39. Yu JC, Lauer MR, Young C, et al. Localization of the origin of the atrioventricular junctional rhythm induced during selective ablation of slow-pathway conduction in patients with atrioventricular-node reentrant tachycardia. Am Heart J. 1996;131:937–46.

40. Wagshal AB, Crystal E, Katz A. Patterns of accelerated junctional rhythm during slow pathway catheter ablation for atrioventricular nodal reentrant tachycardia: temperature dependence, prognostic value, and insights into the nature of the slow pathway. J Cardiovasc Electrophysiol. 2000;11:244–54.

41. Willems S, Shenasa H, Kottkamp H, et al. Temperature-controlled slow pathway ablation for treatment of atrioventricular nodal reentrant tachycardia using a combined anatomical and electrogram guided strategy. Eur Heart J. 1996;17:1092–102.

42. Manolis AS, Wang PJ, Estes NA III. Radiofrequency ablation of slow pathway in patients with atrioventricular nodal reentrant tachycardia. Do arrhythmia recurrences correlate with persistent slow pathway conduction or site of successful ablation? Circulation. 1994;90:2815–19.

43. Rostock T, Risius T, Ventura R, et al. Efficacy and safety of radiofrequency catheter ablation of atrioventricular nodal reentrant tachycardia in the elderly. J Cardiovasc Electrophysiol. 2005;16:608–10.

44. Weismuller P, Kuly S, Brandts B, et al. Is electrical stimulation during administration of catecholamines required for the evaluation of success after ablation of atrioventricular node re-entrant tachycardias? J Am Coll Cardiol. 2002;39:689–94.

45. Stern JD, Aizer A, Rolnitzky L, et al. Meta-analysis to assess the appropriate endpoint for slow pathway ablation of atrioventricular nodal reentrant tachycardia. Pacing Clin Electrophysiol. 2011;34:269–77.

46. Inoue S, Becker A. Posterior extensions of the human compact atrioventricular node: a neglected anatomic feature of potential clinical significance. Circulation. 1998;97:188–93.

47. Anderson RH, Ho SY, Becker AE. Anatomy of the human atrioventricular junctions revisited. Anat Rec. 2000;260:81–91.

48. Waki K, Kim JS, Becker AE. Morphology of the human atrioventricular node is age-dependent: a feature of potential clinical significance. J Cardiovasc Electrophysiol. 2000;1:1144–51.

49. Mazgalev TN, Ho SY, Anderson RH. Anatomic-electrophysiological correlations concerning the pathways for atrioventricular conduction. Circulation. 2001;103:2660–7.

50. Engelstein ED, Stein KM, Markowitz SM, et al. Posterior fast atrioventricular node pathways: Implications for radiofrequency catheter ablation of atrioventricular node reentrant tachycardia. J Am Coll Cardiol. 1996;27:1098–105.

51. Otomo K, Wang Z, Lazzara R, et al. Atrioventricular nodal reentrant tachycardia: electrophysiologic characteristics of four forms and implications for reentrant circuit. In: Zipes D, Jalife J, eds. Cardiac electrophysiology: from cell to bedside. 3rd ed. Philadelphia: WB Saunders; 2000. p. 504–21.

52. Sinkovec M, Pernat A, Rajkovic Z, et al. Electrophysiology of anterograde right-atrial and left-atrial inputs to the atrioventricular node in patients with atrioventricular nodal re-entrant tachycardia. Europace. 2011;13:869–75.

53. Lee KJ, Chun HM, Liem B, et al. Multiple atrioventricular nodal pathways in humans: electrophysiologic demonstration and characterization. J Cardiovasc Electrophysiol. 1998;9:129–40.

54. Heinroth KM, Kattenbeck K, Stabenow I, et al. Multiple AV nodal pathways in patients with AV nodal reentrant tachycardia – more common than expected? Europace. 2002;4:375–82.

55. Thiene G, Wenink A, Frescura C, et al. Surgical anatomy and pathology of the conduction tissues in atrioventricular defects. J Thorac Cardiovasc Surg. 1981;82:928–37.

56. Lin JF, Li YC, Yang PL, et al. Ablation of atrioventricular nodal reentrant tachycardia in a patient with reversal of slow and fast pathways inputs into the

atrioventricular node. Pacing Clin Electrophysiol. 2012;35:e17–e19.

57. Okishige K, Fisher JD, Goseki Y, et al. Radiofrequency catheter ablation for AV nodal reentrant tachycardia associated with persistent left superior vena cava. Pacing Clin Electrophysiol. 1997;20:2213–18.

58. Reithmann C, Hoffmann E, Dorwarth U, et al. Slow pathway ablation in a patient with common AV nodal reentrant tachycardia and complete situs inversus. Europace. 1999;1:283–5.

59. Sakabe K, Fukuda N, Wakayama K, et al. Radiofrequency catheter ablation for atrioventricular nodal reentrant tachycardia in a patient with persistent left superior vena cava. Int J Cardiol. 2004;95:355–7.

60. Ernst S, Ouyang F, Linder C, et al. Modulation of the slow pathway in the presence of a persistent left superior caval vein using the novel magnetic navigation system Niobe. Europace. 2004;6:10–14.

61. Okuyama Y, Oka T, Mizuno H, et al. A case of atrioventricular nodal reentrant tachycardia with atresia of the coronary sinus ostium. Int Heart J. 2005;46: 899–902.

62. Satomi K, Chun J, Bansch D, et al. Catheter ablation of atrioventricular nodal reentrant tachycardia after repair of incomplete endocardial cushion defect. Heart Rhythm. 2007;4:351–4.

63. Sung RJ, Lauer MR. Atrioventricular nodal reentrant tachycardia. In: Sung RJ, Lauer MR, editors. Fundamental approaches to the management of cardiac arrhythmias. Dordrecht: Kluwer Academic Publishers; 2000. pp. 488–509.

64. Silka MJ, Kron J, Park JK, et al. Atypical forms of supraventricular tachycardia due to atrioventricular node reentry in children after radiofrequency modification of slow pathway conduction. J Am Coll Cardiol. 1994;23:1363–9.

65. Kalbfleisch SJ, Strickberger SA, Hummel JD, et al. Double retrograde atrial response after radiofrequency ablation of atypical AV nodal reentrant tachycardia. J Cardiovasc Electrphysiol. 1993;4:695–701.

66. Kay GN, Epstein AE, Dalley SM, et al. A role of radiofrequency ablation in the management of supraventricular arrhythmias: experience in 760 consecutive patients. J Cardiovasc Electrphysiol. 1993;4:371–89.

67. Manolis AS, Wang PJ, Estes NA III. Radiofrequency ablation of slow pathway in patients with atrioventricular nodal reentrant tachycardia: do arrhythmia recurrences correlate with persistent slow pathway conduction or site of successful ablation? Circulation. 1994;90:2815–19.

68. Calkins H, Young P, Miller JM, et al. Catheter ablation of accessory pathways, atrioventricular nodal reentrant tachycardia, and the atrioventricular junction: final results of a prospective, multicenter clinical trial. The Atakr Multicenter Investigators Group. Circulation. 1999;99:262–70.

69. Scheinman MM. NASPE Survey on Catheter Ablation. Pacing Clin Electrophysiol. 1995;18:1474–8.

70. Clague JR, Dagres N, Kottkamp H, et al. Targeting the slow pathway for atrioventricular nodal reentrant tachycardia: initial results and long-term follow-up in 379 consecutive patients. Eur Heart J. 2001;22:82–88.

71. Hoffmann BA, Brachmann J, Andresen D, et al. Ablation of atrioventricular nodal reentrant tachycardia in the elderly: results from the German ablation registry. Heart Rhythm. 2011;8:981–7.

72. Feldman A, Voskoboinik A, Kumar S, et al. Predictors of acute and long-term success of slow pathway ablation for atrioventricular nodal reentrant tachycardia: a single center series of 1,419 consecutive patients. Pacing Clin Electrophysiol. 2011;34:927–33.

73. Fenelon G, d'Avila A, Malacky T, et al. Prognostic significance of transient complete atrioventricular block during radiofrequency ablation of atrioventricular node reentrant tachycardia. Am J Cardiol. 1995;75: 698–702.

74. Kimman GP, Bogaard MD, Vanhemel NM, et al. Ten year follow-up after radiofrequency catheter ablation for atrioventricular nodal reentrant tachycardia in the early days forever cured, or a source for new arrhythmias? Pacing Clin Electrophysiol. 2005;28: 1302–9.

75. Arimoto T, Watanabe T, Nitobe J, et al. Difference of clinical course after catheter ablation of atrioventricular nodal reentrant tachycardia between younger and older patients: atrial vulnerability predicts new onset of atrial fibrillation. Intern Med. 2011;50: 1649–55.

76. Kalusche D, Ott P, Arentz T, et al. AV nodal re-entry tachycardia in elderly patients: clinical presentation and results of radiofrequency catheter ablation therapy. Coron Artery Dis. 1998;9:359–63.

77. Kihel J, Da Costa A, Kihel A, et al. Long-term efficacy and safety of radiofrequency ablation in elderly patients with atrioventricular nodal re-entrant tachycardia. Europace. 2006;8:416–42.

78. Meiltz A, Zimmermann M. Atrioventricular nodal reentrant tachycardia in the elderly: efficacy and safety of radiofrequency catheter ablation. Pacing Clin Electrophysiol. 2007;30:S103–S107.

79. Pedrinazzi C, Durin O, Agricola P, et al. Efficacy and safety of radiofrequency catheter ablation in the elderly. J Interv Card Electrophysiol. 2007;19: 179–85.

80. Haghjoo M, Arya A, Heidari A, et al. Electrophysiologic characteristics and results of radiofrequency catheter ablation in elderly patients with atrioventricular nodal reentrant tachycardia. J Electrocardiol. 2007;40:208–13.

81. Sra JS, Jazayeri MR, Blanck Z, *et al.* Slow pathway ablation in patients with atrioventricular node reentrant tachycardia and a prolonged PR interval. J Am Coll Cardiol. 1994;24:1064–8.

82. Li YG, Gronefeld G, Bender B, *et al.* Risk of development of delayed atrioventricular block after slow pathway modification in patients with atrioventricular nodal reentrant tachycardia and a pre-existing prolonged PR interval. Eur Heart J. 2001;22:89–95.

83. Reithmann C, Remp T, Oversohl N, *et al.* Ablation for atrioventricular nodal reentrant tachycardia with a prolonged PR interval during sinus rhythm: the risk of delayed higher-degree atrioventricular block. J Cardiovasc Electrophysiol. 2006;17:973–9.

84. Pasquie JL, Scalzi J, Macia JC, *et al.* Long-term safety and efficacy of slow pathway ablation in patients with atrioventricular nodal re-entrant tachycardia and pre-existing prolonged PR interval. Europace. 2006; 8:129–33.

85. Schaffer MS, Silka MJ, Ross BA, *et al.* Inadvertent atrioventricular block during radiofrequency catheter ablation: results of the pediatric radiofrequency ablation frequency. Circulation. 1996;94:3214–20.

86. Kugler JD, Danford DA, Deal BJ, *et al.* Radiofrequency catheter ablation for tachyarrhythmias in children and adolescents. The Pediatric Electrophysiology Society. N Engl J Med. 1994;330:1481–7.

87. Kugler JD, Danford DA, Houston KA, *et al.* Radiofrequency catheter ablation for paroxysmal supraventricular tachycardia in children and adolescents without structural heart disease. Pediatric EP Society, Radiofrequency Catheter Ablation Registry. Am J Cardiol. 1997;80:1438–43.

88. Kugler JD, Danford DA, Houston KA, *et al.* Pediatric radiofrequency catheter ablation registry success, fluoroscopy time, and complication rate for supraventricular tachycardia: comparison of early and recent eras. J Cardiovasc Electrophysiol. 2002;13:336–41.

89. Hoffman BF, Cranefield PF. Electrophysiology of the heart. New York: McGraw-Hill; 1960.

90. Thibault B, de Bakker JM, Hocini M, *et al.* Origin of heat-induced accelerated junctional rhythm. J Cardiovasc Electrophysiol. 1998;9:631–41.

91. Inoue S, Becker AE. Koch's triangle sized up: anatomical landmarks in perspective of catheter ablation procedures. Pacing and Clinical Electrophysiology. 1998;21:1553–8.

92. Chauvin M, Shah DC, Haïssaguerre M, *et al.* The anatomic basis of connections between the coronary sinus musculature and the left atrium in humans. Circulation. 2000;101:647–52.

93. Batra R, Nair M, Kumar M, *et al.* Intracardiac echocardiography guided radiofrequency catheter ablation of the slow pathway in atrioventricular nodal reentrant tachycardia. J Interv Cardiac Electrophysiol. 2002;6: 43–9.

94. Kammeraada J, Udink ten Catea F, Simmersa T, *et al.* Radiofrequency catheter ablation of atrioventricular nodal reentrant tachycardia in children aided by the LocaLisa mapping system. Europace. 2004;6: 209–14.

95. Kerst G, Weig HJ, Weretka S, *et al.* Contact force control – the key to safe zero-fluoroscopy catheter ablation of atrioventricular nodal reentrant tachycardia. Dtsch Med Wochenschr. 2011;136:1946–51.

96. Schwagten B, Knops P, Janse P, *et al.* Long-term follow-up after catheter ablation for atrioventricular nodal reentrant tachycardia: a comparison of cryothermal and radiofrequency energy in a large series of patients. J Interv Card Electrophysiol. 2011;30:55–61.

CHAPTER 4

Catheter Cryoablation for Atrioventricular Nodal Reentrant Tachycardia

Ngai-Yin Chan

Princess Margaret Hospital, Hong Kong, China

Atrioventricular nodal reentrant tachycardia (AVNRT) is the commonest form of regular supraventricular tachycardia and accounts for more than 50% of this arrhythmia.[1] Radiofrequency catheter ablation (RFCA) for slow pathway modification or elimination was first described more than 20 years ago.[2–6] High acute procedural success of up to 99% and low recurrence rates of 1–5% have been reported by different studies.[3,4,7–9]

Despite the effectiveness of this treatment, there is a low but genuine risk of inadvertent atrioventricular block (AVB) necessitating permanent pacemaker implantation. The risk of this complication has been reported to vary from 0.4% to 1.3% in earlier studies.[3,4,7,8] In recent years, data have accumulated in the use of catheter cryoablation (CRYO) as an alternative curative treatment for AVNRT. An acute procedural success rate comparable to that of RFCA can be achieved with CRYO. Most importantly, a zero risk of inadvertent AVB may be achievable. However, a higher recurrence rate has been uniformly reported.

In this chapter, the contemporary incidence of inadvertent AVB complicating RFCA for AVNRT, the advantages of CRYO over RFCA in the treatment

of AVNRT, and the strategies to reduce the recurrence rate for patients with AVNRT treated by CRYO are discussed. The techniques of performing CRYO for AVNRT are also detailed.

Atrioventricular block after radiofrequency catheter ablation for atrioventricular nodal reentrant tachycardia

Inadvertent AVB is a known complication of RFCA for AVNRT. However, there is a wide variability of its incidence reported in the literature.[3,4,7,8,10–15] In the seminal work by Jackman et al.,[4] 80 patients with AVNRT underwent RFCA and one (1.3%) patient developed complete heart block and required permanent pacemaker implantation. In a larger prospective multicenter trial reported by Calkins et al.,[10] 5 (1.3%) out of 373 patients with AVNRT were complicated with complete heart block after RFCA. The risk of inadvertent AVB observed in more recent contemporary studies appears much lower. In a large prospective registry involving 3160 patients receiving RFCA for AVNRT, 8 (0.3%) of them developed complete heart block and required

The Practice of Catheter Cryoablation for Cardiac Arrhythmias, First Edition. Edited by Ngai-Yin Chan.
© 2014 John Wiley & Sons, Ltd. Published 2014 by John Wiley & Sons, Ltd.

Table 4.1. Risk of inadvertent atrioventricular block (AVB) complicating radiofrequency ablation of atrioventricular nodal reentrant tachycardia

Authors	Number of patients	Permanent complete AVB	Study design
Jackman et al. (1992)[4]	80	1/80 (1.3%)	Prospective
Calkins et al. (1999)[10]	373	5/373 (1.3%)	Prospective
Clague et al. (2001)[11]	379	3/379 (0.8%)	Retrospective
Hoffmann et al. (2011)[12]	3160	8/3160 (0.3%)	Prospective
Feldman et al. (2011)[13]	1419	1/1419 (0.07%)	Retrospective
Deisenhofer et al. (2010)[14]	258	1/258 (0.4%)	Prospective, randomized, and comparative
Opel et al. (2010)[15]	149	1/149 (0.7%)	Prospective, nonrandomized, and comparative
Schwagten et al. (2011)[30]	124	2/124 (1.6%)	Prospective, nonrandomized, and comparative

permanent pacemaker implantation.[12] Feldman et al.[13] reported only a 0.07% risk of permanent AVB in a retrospective series of 1419 patients undergoing RFCA for AVNRT.

In a nonrandomized comparative study between RFCA and CRYO in the treatment of AVNRT, Opel et al.[15] reported a 0.7% rate of complete heart block in the radiofrequency (RF) arm involving 149 patients. In a recently published randomized comparative study between RFCA and CRYO, Deisenhofer et al.[14] observed that 1 (0.4%) out of 258 patients developed complete heart block after RFCA. The risk of inadvertent AVB complicating RFCA for AVNRT, reported in different representative studies, is summarized in Table 4.1.

The incidence of inadvertent AVB complicating RFCA for AVNRT is likely strongly related to operator experience. The methodology in data collection also affects significantly the reported risk, with anticipated underestimation in retrospective studies. For experienced operators, the expected risk of this complication would be below 1% and varies between 0.3% and 0.7%. For less experienced operators, the expected risk of inadvertent AVB would be close to that reported in the early studies (i.e., around 1.3%).

Is cryoablation free of the complication of permanent inadvertent AVB in the treatment of AVNRT?

There is a theoretical advantage of CRYO over RFCA in minimizing the risk of permanent inadvertent AVB in the treatment of AVNRT. CRYO can produce a more accurate lesion because of its special lesion characteristics, the phenomenon of cryoadhesion, and the ability of cryomapping.

In general, it is believed that CRYO produces a smaller lesion than RFCA.[16] However, it should be better appreciated that this is only an overgeneralized statement. In fact, the lesion volume resulting from CRYO is determined by a multitude of factors, namely, catheter refrigerant flow, convective warming from circulating blood, electrode orientation to tissue, electrode tip size, contact pressure, and finally the temperature reached at the electrode–tissue interface.[17,18] Parvez et al.[18] observed that the lesion volume produced by an 8 mm tip cryocatheter can be smaller or larger than that of an open irrigated radiofrequency (RF) ablation catheter (Figure 4.1).[18]

The stability of the catheter is enhanced by the phenomenon of cryoadhesion for CRYO. The tip of the cryocatheter adheres to the cardiac tissue when the temperature reaches −30 °C or below. *Cryomapping* refers to the ability to achieve reversible electrophysiological effects when the temperature of the catheter tip is lowered to −30 °C.[19] This improves significantly the safety of CRYO compared to RFCA, especially in terms of prevention of permanent inadvertent AVB.

Since the prevalence of permanent inadvertent AVB in RFCA for AVNRT is low, a large randomized comparative study will be needed to test the hypothesis that an even lower or zero risk of this complication can be achieved by CRYO. To date, there has

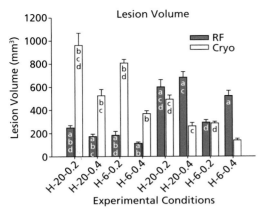

Figure 4.1. A Comparison in lesion volume created by radiofrequency with a 3.5 mm saline-irrigated catheter (red bars) and cryoablation with an 8 mm catheter (white bars) under different conditions. H: horizontal catheter orientation; V: vertical catheter orientation; 0.2: 0.2 m/s blood velocity; 0.4: 0.4 m/s blood velocity; 6: 6 g contact pressure; 20: 20 g contact pressure. (Source: Adapted from Parvez B, Pathak V, Schubert CM, et al, 2008[18]. Reproduced with permission from John Wiley and Sons Ltd).

been no such study performed to address this fundamental question. However, with over a decade of experience, the hypothesis that CRYO for AVNRT carries zero risk of permanent inadvertent AVB gets closer and closer to reality. There has not been a single reported case of this complication in using CRYO to treat AVNRT. More importantly, no patient suffered from this complication in the CRYO arm in all the published comparative studies between CRYO and RFCA for treating AVNRT (Table 4.2). In contrast, 0.9% of patients in the RFCA arm suffered from this complication, and 0.5% of patients required implantation of permanent pacemakers.

Other advantages of using cryoablation to treat AVNRT

One notable feature and advantage of CRYO is that it is painless or significantly less painful than RFCA. Instead of stimulating the afferent pain fibers in the myocardium as in RFCA, CRYO freezes and inactivates them.[26] CRYO has been shown to be less

Table 4.2. Prevalence of permanent inadvertent atrioventricular block (AVB) in comparative studies of cryoablation (CRYO) and radiofrequency catheter ablation (RFCA) for atrioventricular nodal reentrant tachycardia (AVNRT)

Authors	Radiofrequency arm (N)	Permanent inadvertent AVB complicating RFCA			CRYO arm (N)	Permanent inadvertent AVB complicating CRYO
		First degree	Second degree	Third degree		
Kimman *et al.* (2004)[20]	33	0	0	0	30	0
Zrenner *et al.* (2004)[21]	100	1	0	0	100	0
Collins *et al.* (2006)[22]	60	0	0	0	57	0
Gupta *et al.* (2006)[25]	71	0	1	0	71	0
Avari *et al.* (2008)[23]	42	0	0	0	38	0
Chan *et al.* (2009)[24]	80	1	1	0	80	0
Opel *et al.* (2010)[15]	149	0	0	1	123	0
Deisenhofer *et al.* (2010)[14]	258	2	0	1	251	0
Schwagten *et al.* (2011)[30]	124	0	0	2	150	0
Total	917	4	2	2	900	0

painful than RFCA in the treatment of atrial flutter.[27] RFCA has also been shown to be painful in the treatment of supraventricular arrhythmias, including AVNRT.[28] In a small randomized comparative study by Chan et al.,[29] patients treated with CRYO for AVNRT experienced significantly less pain than those treated with RFCA. This was subsequently confirmed in a larger randomized comparative study by Deisenhofer et al.[14]

Continuous and vigorous surveillance of the catheter position by fluoroscopy and intracardiac electrograms is of utmost importance in RFCA for AVNRT. This may generate significant operator stress. It has been shown in a small randomized comparative study that CRYO creates significantly less operator stress than RFCA in the treatment of AVNRT.[29] Because CRYO creates a smaller lesion and has the properties of cryoadhesion and cryomapping, the operator may perceive himself or herself to be in better control of the procedure.

The operators may reduce the fluoroscopic screening of ablation catheter position during CRYO because of the phenomenon of cryoadhesion. In contrast, continuous fluoroscopy is in general recommended for RFCA. There is a discordance of results in terms of fluoroscopy time in different comparative studies between CRYO and RFCA for AVNRT. In general, most of the studies show either a shorter[21,24,30] or similar[14,20,22,23,25] fluoroscopy time with CRYO compared with the RFCA arm.

Recurrence rates: The Achilles' Heel of cryoablation in treating AVNRT

A high acute procedural success rate for AVNRT ablation can be achieved with CRYO. In general, an acute procedural success rate of >95% can be achieved with either a 4 mm or 6 mm tip cryocatheter, and it is comparable to that of RFCA (Table 4.3).[14,15,20–25,30] However, there is a consistently higher recurrence rate in patients receiving CRYO for treating AVNRT. The recurrence rate varies from 3% to 20% when 4 mm tip cryocatheters were used.[20–23,25,30] A larger 6 mm tip cryocatheter was tested in subsequent studies.[14,15,24] Disappointingly, despite higher uniformity, the recurrence rate is 9–10% and is still significantly higher than that of RFCA.

The comparably high acute procedural success rate, yet higher recurrence rate, of CRYO compared to RFCA in the treatment of AVNRT is likely related to the biophysical properties of cryolesion. During CRYO, the frozen tissue is characterized by a central zone of intracellular freezing with cell death, and a peripheral zone of extracellular freezing with transient and incomplete cellular injury.[31] Interestingly, only less than 30% of the frozen tissue is included in the −40 °C isotherm, which is believed to be a temperature necessary for creation of a permanent cryolesion. The high recurrence rate of AVNRT treated by CRYO is probably due to delayed recovery of the peripheral zone of the cryolesion.

Table 4.3. Comparison of acute procedural success and recurrence rate between catheter cryoablation (CRYO) and radiofrequency catheter ablation (RFCA) in the treatment of atrioventricular nodal reentrant tachycardia

| Authors | Acute procedural success rate | | | Recurrence rate | | | |
	Radiofrequency (RF) (%)	Cryo (%)	p value	RF (%)	Cryo (%)	P value	Cryocatheter size (mm)
Kimman et al. (2004)[20]	91	93	NS	10	11	NS	4
Zrenner et al. (2004)[21]	98	97	NS	1	8	0.017	4
Collins et al. (2006)[22]	100	95	NS	2	8	NS	4
Gupta et al. (2006)[25]	97	85	<0.01	6	20	0.01	4 and 6
Avari et al. (2008)[23]	95	97	NS	2	3	NS	4 and 6
Chan et al. (2009)[24]	95	98	NS	1	9	0.032	6
Opel et al. (2010)[15]	95	93	NS	3	10	0.02	6
Deisenhofer et al. (2010)[14]	98	97	NS	4	9	0.029	6
Schwagten et al. (2011)[30]	96	96	NS	5	11	NS	4

NS: nonsignificant.

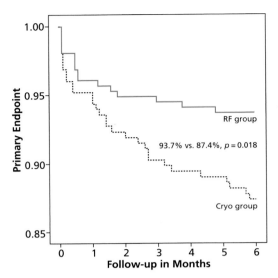

Figure 4.2. A Kaplan–Meier curve showing the difference in the composite primary endpoint of procedural failure, recurrence, and atrioventricular block. Cryo: catheter cryoablation; RF: radio frequency catheter ablation. (Source: Adapted from Deisenhofer I, Zrenner B, Yin YH, et al, 2010[14]. Reproduced with permission from Wolters Kluwer Health).

To compare the performance of CRYO and RFCA in the treatment of AVNRT, a composite including acute procedural failure, permanent AVB, and recurrence is a very useful endpoint. In the Cryoablation versus Radiofrequency Energy for the Ablation of Atrioventricular Nodal Reentrant Tachycardia (CYRANO) study, CRYO with a 6 mm cryocatheter has been shown to be inferior to RFCA with respect to this composite endpoint (Figure 4.2).[14]

Procedural techniques of cryoablation for AVNRT

See Video Clip 4.1.

Baseline electrophysiology study

The basic setup for a diagnostic electrophysiology study of CRYO is similar to that of RFCA, with four electrode catheters positioned to the right atrium, His bundle, coronary sinus and right ventricular apex, respectively. Incremental atrial and ventricular pacing and extrastimulus testing from the right atrium and right ventricle are performed. If sus-

tained tachycardia cannot be induced, isoprenalin can be infused to facilitate tachycardia induction. Dual AV nodal physiology is identified by a sudden AH jump or HA jump of at least 50 ms in response to programmed atrial or ventricular extrastimulation. AV nodal reentrant tachycardia is diagnosed on the basis of standard criteria.[32] For the purpose of cryomapping, the baseline PR and AH interval, the atrioventricular Wenckebach cycle length, the effective refractory periods of fast pathway and slow pathway, and the induction protocol that reproducibly demonstrates dual AV nodal physiology and induces AVNRT are of particular importance.

Target sites for cryoablation

Similar to RFCA, the target site for ablating AVNRT with cryothermic energy is in the triangle of Koch. A combination of electrogram and anatomical approaches adopted from experience in RFCA[33] is commonly described in the literature on CRYO for AVNRT. However, the most optimal amplitude ratio of the atrial and ventricular signals at the target site has not been studied for CRYO. In general, a ratio of 0.25–0.5 is recommended. In the author's experience, the successful ablation site usually associates with a small-amplitude atrial electrogram with "slow pathway potential" evidenced by double potentials or fractionated electrograms and a large-amplitude ventricular electrogram. It should also be well appreciated that the most optimal amplitude ratio may be variable among different patients, especially when larger 6 mm or 8 mm tip cryocatheters are used.

The anatomical region between the ostium of the coronary sinus and the bundle of His can be divided into six equally spaced parts, namely, P1, P2, M1, M2, A1, and A2 from posteriorly to anteriorly.[32] Chan *et al.*[29] has shown in a small randomized study that the proportion of posteriorly located targeted ablation sites (P1 or P2) was significantly higher in the RFCA group than in the CRYO group (Table 4.4). This observation may reflect that the operator deliberately stayed away from more anterior locations with RFCA to avoid inadvertent AVB, or one may hypothesize that the optimal ablation site for CRYO is quite often in the M1 or M2 regions.

Cryomapping

The function of cryomapping can be performed by lowering the catheter tip temperature to −30 °C,

Table 4.4. Targeted ablation sites in a randomized study comparing catheter cryoablation (CRYO) with radiofrequency catheter ablation (RFCA) for atrioventricular nodal reentrant tachycardia. (Source: Adapted from Chan NY, Choy CC, Lau CL, et al, 2011[44]. Reproduced with permission from John Wiley and Sons Ltd).

	CRYO (n = 104)	RFCA (n = 72)	P value
P1 or P2	59	52	0.036
M1 or M2	40	20	—
A1 or A2	5	0	—

P1, P2, M1, M2, A1, and A2: six equally spaced regions from below the ostium of coronary sinus posteriorly to the bundle of His anteriorly.

and it is available for both 4 mm and 6 mm tip cryocatheters. Transient electrophysiological effect will occur and full recovery of electrophysiological function is expected with rewarming within 60 s. At any potential ablation site, the catheter tip temperature is lowered to −30 °C for a maximal duration of 60 s to test the electrophysiological effect by using programmed electrical stimulation that has reproducibly demonstrated dual AV nodal physiology or induced AVNRT. If cryomapping at a potential site resulted in no desirable electrophysiological effect or AVB, cryomapping can be stopped and repeated at a new target site (Figure 4.3). Elimination of slow pathway and noninducibility of AVNRT are commonly regarded as endpoints for successful cryomapping. However, in the author's experience, elimination of slow pathway is a much preferred endpoint for cryomapping in AVNRT (Figure 4.4).

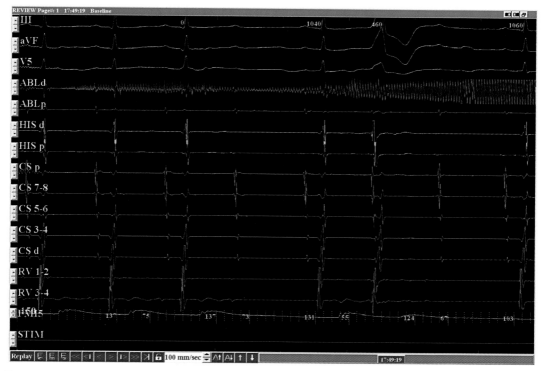

Figure 4.3. Atrioventricular block that occurred during cryoablation, despite the absence of this complication during cryomapping. Cryoablation was stopped, and normal atrioventricular conduction resumed within a few seconds.

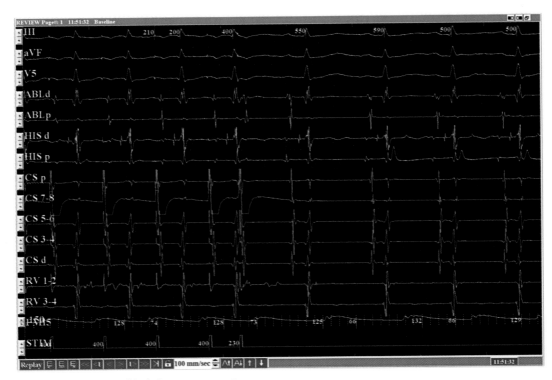

Figure 4.4. Slow pathway block during cryomapping.

A short time-to-effect of 10–20 s is an indicator for an appropriate ablation site. Usually, a change in the AV Wenckebach cycle length is observed. It has to be emphasized that surveillance for AVB is also necessary during cryoablation since this complication can still occur even with prior successful cryomapping.[20,21] In the author's experience, an increase of >20–25% of the PR or AH intervals should alert the operator to stop cryomapping or cryoablation and search for another target site.

Cryoablation protocol

After successful cryomapping, the catheter tip temperature is lowered to −75 °C to −80 °C for cryoablation. A 4 min cycle is commonly used. Double freezing with two 4 min cycles may be used at the same or nearly the same ablation site to increase lesion size and depth. The use of a linear lesion approach by sequential ablation of sites with different amplitude ratios of the atrial and ventricular electrograms in the triangle of Koch has also been described.[34] After initial success with cryoablation, repeat testing for early recurrence after 30 min is highly recommended.

Strategies to decrease the recurrence rate after cryoablation for AVNRT

A more robust ablation endpoint

The most appropriate endpoint for AVNRT ablation remains unclear for both RFCA and CRYO. A good balance among inadvertent AVB, recurrence rate, and procedural time is the crux. The commonly used endpoints in RFCA include slow pathway elimination with disappearance of dual nodal physiology, and slow pathway modification with either residual dual nodal physiology without AV nodal echo beat or dual nodal physiology with up to one AV nodal echo beat.

Whether elimination of slow pathway is necessary for RFCA of AVNRT remains controversial. Estner et al. studied 506 consecutive patients with AVNRT who underwent RFCA.[35] There was a recurrence rate of 5.2%, and it was not predicted by slow pathway elimination. In contrast, a meta-analysis including 10 studies with 1204 patients showed that a significantly higher recurrence rate occurred in patients with residual dual nodal physiology with or without a single AV nodal echo beat, when isoproterenol was used after ablation for testing if it is only needed to induce AVNRT before ablation.[36] Feldman *et al.* reported their observation in a single-center series of 1419 patients with AVNRT and RFCA.[37] There was a 1.5% recurrence rate, and the presence of residual dual nodal physiology with or without one AV nodal echo beat was not predictive of recurrence. However, patients with a single AV nodal echo beat and recurrence had a significantly wider echo window (85 ms) than patients without recurrence (30 ms).

In CRYO for AVNRT, the commonly used endpoint reported in randomized or nonrandomized studies was slow pathway modification with residual dual nodal physiology. An AV nodal echo beat was usually accepted as an ablation endpoint. There have been increasing data recently reported on the superiority of using slow pathway elimination as the endpoint of CRYO for AVNRT. Gupta *et al.* observed in a retrospective series of 71 patients that the recurrence rate after CRYO for AVNRT was significantly higher if an AV nodal echo beat was still inducible after ablation than if slow pathway elimination was achieved.[25] In a prospective series of 160 patients, Sandilands *et al.* reported that a lower recurrence rate after CRYO for AVNRT could be achieved if a 6 mm instead of a 4 mm tip cryocatheter was used and slow pathway elimination was confirmed after ablation.[38] In line with these two studies, Eckhardt *et al.* achieved a low recurrence rate of 4% after CRYO for AVNRT in 75 patients by using an ablation endpoint of elimination of tachycardia plus AH jump with one AV nodal echo beat.[39] However, in a single center cohort of 185 patients

with AVNRT who underwent CRYO, independent predictors of recurrence were only younger age and valvular heart disease, but not persistent AV nodal physiology with or without AV nodal echo beat.[40]

Use of an 8 mm tip cryocatheter

Increasing the lesion size of CRYO is a potential strategy to reduce the recurrence rate after AVNRT treatment. The size of a cryolesion is dependent on multiple factors, including local blood flow, electrode orientation, electrode contact pressure, and electrode size.[17] Since the use of a 6 mm tip cryocatheter in the treatment of AVNRT still resulted in a higher recurrence rate compared with RFCA,[14,24] this led to the attempt to use an 8 mm tip cryocatheter in AVNRT ablation. Under favorable catheter orientation, contact pressure, and local blood flow, the lesion created by an 8 mm tip cryocatheter may be even larger than that created by a 3.5 mm tip saline-irrigated RF catheter[18] (Figure 4.1). Silver *et al.* reported their initial experience of using an 8 mm tip cryocatheter to treat 77 pediatric patients with AVNRT.[41] They achieved an acute procedural success rate of 91% and only 2.8% recurrence rate with a mean follow-up period of 11.6 months. There was no complication of inadvertent AVB. In a small retrospective case–control study performed by Chan *et al.*,[42] 20 patients with AVNRT treated with an 8 mm cryocatheter were compared with 20 patients treated with RFCA (Figure 4.5). Treatment failure was defined as the composite of acute procedural failure including inadvertent permanent AVB and documented recurrence. There was no significant difference between the two treatment groups

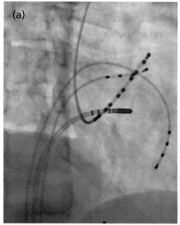 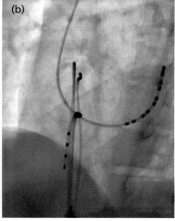

Figure 4.5. Use of an 8 mm tip cryocatheter for AVNRT ablation.
(a) Right anterior oblique (RAO) view.
(b) Left anterior oblique (LAO) view.

in terms of acute procedural success (CRYO 90% vs. RFCA 95%; $p = 0.998$), recurrence rate (CRYO 5.6% vs. RFCA 0%; $p = 0.304$), or treatment failure (CRYO 15% vs. RFCA 5%; $p = 0.301$). A large-scale randomized study comparing CYRO with an 8 mm tip catheter and RFCA in patients with AVNRT is currently underway (the Comparative Study between Cryoablation and Radiofrequency Ablation in the Treatment of Supraventricular Tachycardia [CRYO-ABLATE] study).[43] It may shed more light on this very important issue in using CRYO to treat AVNRT.

Conclusions

Radiofrequency has been the primary source of energy for AVNRT ablation. The acute procedural success rate is high, and the recurrence rate is low. However, there is a low risk of inadvertent AVB necessitating pacemaker implantation even with experienced operators. Cryoablation is an alternative approach to treat AVNRT, and it may eliminate the risk of inadvertent AVB. Other advantages of CRYO include less patient pain perception, less operator stress, and decrease in fluoroscopic exposure. The current challenge of CRYO is the high recurrence rate. The use of a more robust ablation endpoint of slow pathway elimination and the use of an 8 mm cryocatheter are two promising strategies to reduce the recurrence rate.

 Interactive Case Studies related to this chapter can be found at this book's companion website, at **www.chancryoablation.com**

References

1. Porter MJ, Morton JB, Denman R, *et al.* Influence of age and gender on the mechanism of supraventricular tachycardia. Heart Rhythm. 2004;1:393–6.

2. Lee MA, Morady F, Kadish A, *et al.* Catheter modification of the atrioventricular junction with radiofrequency energy for control of atrioventricular nodal reentry tachycardia. Circulation. 1991;83:827–35.

3. Haissaguerre M, Gaita F, Fischer B, *et al.* Elimination of atrioventricular nodal re-entrant tachycardia using discrete slow potentials to guide application of radiofrequency energy. Circulation. 1992;85: 2162–75.

4. Jackman WM, Beckman KJ, McClelland JH, *et al.* Treatment of supraventricular tachycardia due to atrioventricular nodal reentry, by radiofrequency catheter ablation of slow-pathway conduction. N Engl J Med. 1992;327:313–8.

5. Jazayeri MR, Hempe SL, Sra JS, *et al.* Selective transcatheter ablation of the fast and slow pathways using radiofrequency energy in patients with atrioventricular nodal reentrant tachycardia. Circulation. 1992;85:1318–28.

6. Kay GN, Epstein AE, Dailey SM, *et al.* Selective radiofrequency ablation of the slow pathway for the treatment of atrioventricular nodal reentrant tachycardia. Evidence for involvement of perinodal myocardium within the re-entrant circuit. Circulation. 1992;85: 1675–88.

7. Scheinman MM, Yang Y. The history of AV nodal reentry. Pacing Clin Electrophysiol. 2005;28: 1232–7.

8. Morady F. Catheter ablation of supraventricular arrhythmias: state of the art. Pacing Clin Electrophysiol. 2004;27:125–42.

9. Heidbuchel H. How to ablate typical "slow/fast" AV nodal reentry tachycardia. Europace. 2000;2:15–9.

10. Calkins H, Yong P, Miller JM, *et al.* Catheter ablation of accessory pathways, atrioventricular nodal reentrant tachycardia and the atrioventricular junction: final results of a prospective, multicenter clinical trial. Circulation. 1999;99:262–70.

11. Clague JR, Dagres N, Kottkamp H, *et al.* Targeting the slow pathway for atrioventricular nodal reentrant tachycardia: initial results and long-term follow-up in 379 consecutive patients. Eur Heart J. 2001;22: 82–8.

12. Hoffmann BA, Brachmann J, Andresen D, *et al.* Ablation of atrioventricular nodal reentrant tachycardia in the elderly: results from the German Ablation Registry. Heart. 2011;8:981–7.

13. Feldman A, Voskoboinik A, Kumar S, *et al.* Predictors of acute and long-term success of slow pathway ablation for atrioventricular nodal re-entrant tachycardia: a single centre series of 1419 consecutive patients. Pacing Clin Electrophysiol. 2011;34:927–33.

14. Deisenhofer I, Zrenner B, Yin YH, *et al.* Cryoablation versus radiofrequency energy for the ablation of atrioventricular nodal reentrant tachycardia (the CYRANO study). Results from a large multicenter prospective randomized trial. Circulation. 2010;122: 2239–45.

15. Opel A, Murray S, Kamath N, *et al.* Cryoablation versus radiofrequency ablation for treatment of atrioventricular nodal re-entrant tachycardia: cryoablation with 6-mm-tip catheter is still less effective than radiofrequency ablation. Heart Rhythm. 2010;7:340–3.

16. Rodriguez LM, Leunissen J, Hoekstra A, *et al.* Transvenous cold mapping and cryoablation of the AV node in dogs: observations of chronic lesions and comparison to those obtained with radiofrequency ablation. J Cardiovasc Electrophysiol. 1998;9: 1055–61.

17. Wood MA, Parvez B, Ellenbogen AL, *et al.* Determinants of lesion sizes and tissue temperatures during catheter cryoablation. Pacing Clin Electrophysiol. 2007;30:644–54.

18. Parvez B, Pathak V, Schubert CM, *et al.* Comparison of lesion sizes produced by cryoablation and open irrigation radiofrequency ablation catheters. J Cardiovasc Electrophysiol. 2008;19:528–34.

19. Friedman PL, Dubuc M, Green MS, *et al.* Catheter cryoablation of supraventricular tachycardia: results of the multicenter prospective "frosty" trial. Heart Rhythm. 2004;1:129–38.

20. Kimman GP, Theuns DAMJ, Szili-Torok T, *et al.* CRAVT: a prospective, randomized study comparing transvenous cryothermal and radiofrequency ablation in atrioventricular nodal re-entrant tachycardia. Eur Heart J. 2004;25:2232–7.

21. Zrenner B, Dong J, Schreieck J, *et al.* Transvenous cryoablation versus radiofrequency ablation of the slow pathway for the treatment of atrioventricular nodal reentrant tachycardia: a prospective randomized pilot study. Eur Heart J. 2004;25:2226–31.

22. Collins KK, Dubin AM, Chiesa NA, *et al.* Cryoablation versus radiofrequency ablation for treatment of paediatric atrioventricular nodal re-entrant tachycardia: initial experience with 4-mm cryocatheter. Heart Rhythm. 2006;3:564–70.

23. Avari JN, Jay KS, Rhee EK. Experience and results during transition from radiofrequency ablation to cryoablation for treatment of paediatric atrioventricular nodal re-entrant tachycardia. Pacing Clin Electrophysiol. 2008;31:454–60.

24. Chan NY, Mok NS, Lau CL, *et al.* Treatment of atrioventricular nodal reentrant tachycardia by cryoablation with a 6mm-tip catheter versus radiofrequency ablation. Europace. 2009;11:1065–70.

25. Gupta D, Al-lamee RK, Earley MJ, *et al.* Cryoablation compared with radiofrequency ablation for atrioventricular nodal re-entrant tachycardia: analysis of factors contributing to acute and follow-up outcome. Europace. 2006;8:1022–6.

26. Randall WC, Ardell JL. Functional anatomy of the cardiac efferent innervation. In: Kulbertus HE, Franck G, editors. Neurocardiology. Mount Kisco, NY: Futura; 1988. p. 3–24.

27. Timmermans C, Aeyers GM, Crijins HJ, *et al.* Randomized study comparing radiofrequency ablation with cryoablation for the treatment of atrial flutter with emphasis on pain perception. Circulation. 2003;107:1250–2.

28. Lowe MD, Meara M, Mason J, *et al.* Catheter cryoablation of supraventricular arrhythmias: a painless alternative to radiofrequency energy. Pacing Clin Electrophysiol. 2003;26(1 Pt. 2):500–3.

29. Chan NY, Choy CC, Lau CL, *et al.* Cryoablation versus radiofrequency ablation for atrioventricular nodal re-entrant tachycardia: patient pain perception and operator stress. Pacing Clin Electrophysiol. 2011;34: 2–7.

30. Schwagten B, Knops P, Janse P, *et al.* Long-term follow-up after catheter ablation for atrioventricular nodal re-entrant tachycardia: a comparison of cryothermal and radiofrequency energy in a large series of patients. J Interv Card Electrophysiol. 2011;30: 55–61.

31. Gage AA, Snyder KK, Baust JM, *et al.* The principles of cryobiology: In Dubuc M, Khairy P, editors. Cryoablation for cardiac arrhythmias. Montreal: Vision Commun; 2008. p. 3–12.

32. Jackman WM. Three forms of atrioventricular nodal (junctional) re-entrant tachycardia: differential diagnosis, electrophysiological characteristics, and implications for anatomy of the re-entrant circuit. In: Zipes DP, Jalife J, editors. Cardiac electrophysiology: from cell to bedside. Philadelphia, PA: WB Saunders; 1995. p. 620–37.

33. Kalbfleisch SJ, Strickberger SA, Williamson B, *et al.* Randomized comparison of anatomic and electrogram approaches to ablation of the slow pathway of atrioventricular nodal re-entrant tachycardia. J Am Coll Cardiol. 1994;23:716–23.

34. Czosek RJ, Anderson J, Marino B, *et al.* Linear lesion cryoablation for the treatment of atrioventricular nodal re-entrant tachycardia in paediatrics and young adults. Pacing Clin Electrophysiol. 2010;33: 1304–11.

35. Estner HL, Ndrepera G, Dong J, *et al.* Acute and long-term results of slow pathway ablation in patients with atrioventricular nodal reentrant tachycardia – an analysis of the predictive factors for arrhythmia recurrence. Pacing Clin Electrophysiol. 2005;28:102–10.

36. Stern JD, Rolnitzky L, Goldberg J, *et al.* Meta-analysis to assess the appropriate endpoint for slow pathway ablation of atrioventricular nodal reentrant tachycardia. Pacing Clin Electrophysiol. 2011;34:269–77.

37. Feldman A, Voskoboinik A, Kumar S, *et al.* Predictors of acute and long-term success of slow pathway ablation for atrioventricular nodal re-entrant tachycardia: a single center series of 1,419 consecutive patients. Pacing Clin Electrophysiol. 2011;34:927–33.

38. Sandilands A, Boreham P, Pitts-Crick J, *et al.* Impact of cryoablation catheter size on success rates in the

treatment of atrioventricular nodal reentry tachycardia in 160 patients with long-term follow-up. Europace. 2008;10:683–6.

39. Eckhardt LLL, Leal M, Hollis Z, *et al.* Cryoablation for AVNRT: importance of ablation endpoint criteria. J Cardiovasc Electrophysiol. 2012;23:729–34.

40. Khairy P, Novak PG, Guerra PG, *et al.* Cryothermal slow pathway modification for atrioventricular nodal re-entrant tachycardia. Europace. 2007;9:909–14.

41. Silver ES, Silva JNA, Ceresnak SR, *et al.* Cryoablation with an 8-mm tip catheter for pediatric atrioventricular nodal reentrant tachycardia is safe and efficacious with a low incidence of recurrence. Pacing Clin Electrophysiol. 2010;33:681–6.

42. Chan NY, Mok NS, Choy CC, *et al.* Treatment of atrioventricular nodal re-entrant tachycardia by cryoablation with an 8-mm tip catheter versus radiofrequency ablation. J Interv Card Electrophysiol. 2012;34: 295–301.

43. ClinicalTrials.gov. Comparative Study between Cryoablation and Radiofrequency Ablation in the Treatment of Supraventricular Tachycardia (CRYO-ABLATE). ClinicalTrials.gov ID: NCT01584154. http://clinicaltrials.gov/ct2/show/NCT01584154

CHAPTER 5

Cryoballoon Pulmonary Vein Isolation for Atrial Fibrillation

Jürgen Vogt

Ruhr University Bochum, Bad Oeynhausen, Germany

Introduction

Ostial segmental pulmonary vein ablation was first introduced by Michel Haissaguerre.[1] It was associated with a high rate of reconnection of the pulmonary veins to the atrium (i.e., a high recurrence rate in patients with paroxysmal atrial fibrillation).[2] Additional complications include fibrosis and scarring, ultimately leading to pulmonary vein stenosis or even occlusion. Neither surgery nor other interventions are capable of fully restoring a completely normal pulmonary vein anatomy in such cases.

Comparing cryoablation with radiofrequency (RF) ablation experimentally revealed that the former preserves the extracellular matrix and causes only minor thrombus formation. In addition, cryolesions are more homogeneous and not associated with intimal disruption. Pulmonary vein cryoablation was not expected to cause pulmonary vein stenosis.[3]

Since the turn of the millennium, cryothermal techniques became the preferred approach to pulmonary vein isolation, and the methods underwent further refinements. Using 4 mm and 6 mm catheter tips and nitrous oxide as a refrigerant in conjunction with the Lasso catheter technique, pulmonary vein isolation could be performed without complications. Yet the recurrence rate remained high, and the long duration of each freezing cycle prolonged the procedure time. Introduction of a 9 French catheter with an 8 mm cryotip (Freezor Max) was the next refinement. In segmental ablation, an immediate effect on the myocardial sleeves became evident. Pulmonary vein antral isolation by means of Freezor™ Max was impossible.

Aiming for a single-shot strategy, CryoCath Canada (now Medtronic CryoCath, QB, Canada) developed a spiral curvilinear cryocatheter with self-expanding properties, the Arctic Circler™. Expansion of the catheter from a diameter of 18 mm to 25 mm during cooling was supposed to create a contiguous lesion encircling the pulmonary vein antrum. Since the pulmonary veins are often rather large and mostly funnel shaped, lesions at the pulmonary vein ostium turned out to be noncontiguous. To achieve ostial isolation, the catheter had to be rotated to create several overlapping linear lesions. Isolation was unreliable, however. A large percentage of patients developed recurrent atrial fibrillation. Nevertheless, pulmonary vein

The Practice of Catheter Cryoablation for Cardiac Arrhythmias, First Edition. Edited by Ngai-Yin Chan.
© 2014 John Wiley & Sons, Ltd. Published 2014 by John Wiley & Sons, Ltd.

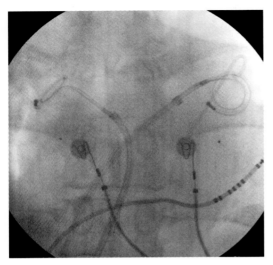

Figure 5.1. Double Arctic Circler simultaneously controlled by two consoles.

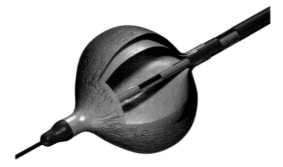

Figure 5.2. Double-layer balloon for safety reasons. (Reproduced with permission of Medtronic, Inc.)

stenoses were never seen after these systematic cryoablation cycles. At the Heart Center North Rhine-Westphalia, procedure and fluoroscopy times were halved by treating two contralateral pulmonary veins simultaneously from two consoles and with two catheters (Figure 5.1; and see Video Clip 5.1).

For treating the pulmonary vein antrum with a single-shot strategy independent of the particular anatomy, the steerable cryoballoon Arctic Front™ (Medtronic CryoCath) was developed in 2005 with both 23 mm and 28 mm balloon diameters.

Function of the Arctic Front cryoballoon

For safety reasons, the Arctic Front cryoballoon is double walled (Figure 5.2). After inflation and positioning, nitrous oxide is delivered via an injection tube and reaches the injectors in each of the balloon's four quadrants from where it is equatorially distributed. Refrigerant leaks are carefully avoided by vacuum-controlled balloon layers and by the balloon walls being attached at offset positions on the catheter shaft. Vaporized nitrous oxide is vacuumed back into the console. The temperature in the proximal balloon is monitored by a thermocouple. Refrigerant flow, pressure, and temperature as well as cooling and rewarming curves are displayed on the control console (Figure 5.3).

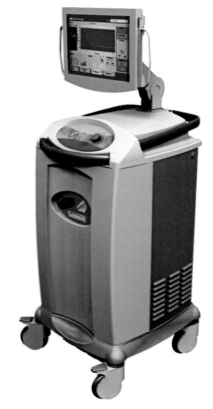

Figure 5.3. Console. (Reproduced with permission of Medtronic, Inc.)

Two pull-wires, which are very proximally attached, allow bilateral balloon deflection. Being an over-the-wire balloon with a 10.5 French outer diameter, the catheter is maneuvered into the left atrium through a Flexcath™ sheath (Medtronic CryoCath)

(a)   (b)

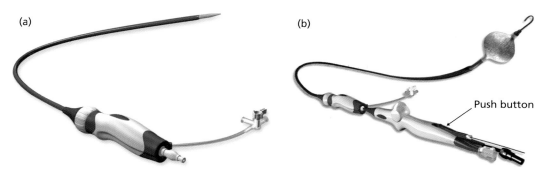

Push button

Figure 5.4. (a) Flexcath™ sheath with inner dilator. (b) Flexcath sheath with balloon in place. Push button. (Both images reproduced with permission of Medtronic, Inc.)

with a 12 French inner and a 15 French outer diameter before it is advanced far into a pulmonary vein over a 0.032–0.035 inch stiff wire or an inner-lumen circular mapping catheter, the Achieve™ catheter (Medtronic CryoCath). After de-airing, the sheath and the balloon's wire lumen are flushed continuously in order to avoid air embolism.

Ablation of the pulmonary vein antrum – technique

See Video Clip 5.2. Balloon positioning at the pulmonary vein ostium is primarily accomplished by deflection of the Flexcath sheath (Figure 5.4a). When the balloon is in position at the pulmonary vein, it is inflated without pressure and tightly held against the pulmonary vein ostium in line with the guidewire. Occlusion is checked by manually injecting diluted contrast agent into the guidewire lumen. Optimally, no contrast agent should reflux. The balloon may not be advanced too far into the vein, a position easily recognized by the oval-shaped balloon silhouette becoming compressed. When the balloon is optimally positioned at the vein antrum, refrigerant delivery commences. The high pressure in the balloon causes the outer balloon shape to change slightly; it becomes more oval and slightly larger. This can make the balloon tilt or slide backward. Even a small positional change can lead to incomplete occlusion and to the balloon temperature not dropping to the lowest value possible. After 4 to 6 min of freezing, balloon rewarming is initiated from the console. When reaching 20 °C, the balloon is automatically deflated. When the push button at the catheter handle is activated, the

balloon tip is extended, folding itself more tightly around the shaft so that it can be retracted into the Flexcath sheath without resistance (Figure 5.4b).

Significance of measuring the proximal balloon temperature

Measured temperatures depend on balloon size and surface area. First, during refrigerant delivery, the measured temperature drops to a lower value in the 23 mm than in the 28 mm balloon. Second, increased balloon surface contact with the vein or atrial wall and less exposure of the balloon surface to flowing blood translate to lower temperatures. The third factor is the extent of occlusion for the temperature that will be ultimately reached. No clear target temperatures are defined, however, because individual anatomical variations of the vein antrum as well as the cardiac output affect external warming of the balloon. Very high temperatures (>−30 °C) could be indicative of insufficient occlusion. Very low temperatures (<−70 °C) should raise suspicion that the balloon may have slipped too far into the pulmonary vein. Proper balloon placement needs to be verified in both cases.

Factors determining lesion size and homogeneity

Lesion size depends on a rapid cooling rate of 20 to 50 °C per min. It is also determined by the lowest tissue temperatures reached. Persistent cooling over a time frame of 4 to 5 min is a prerequisite for the formation of a complete transmural lesion. Delayed rewarming causes recrystallization and destroys the microcirculation, homogenizing the lesion. Repetitive freezing and rewarming cycles enlarge the zone of tissue necrosis. The use of at least two freezes per vein is an important cryobiophysical principle.[4] In animal experiments, a freezing duration of 4 min was found to be ideal.[5] Specifics of the human anatomy need to be taken into account, however, especially the significantly higher tissue thickness at the border zone between the superior veins and the roof of the left atrium and the ridge as well as inferiorly in the vicinity of the carina between ipsilateral veins, particularly in hypertrophied hearts. A freezing duration of 4 to 6 min and repeated freeze-thaw cycles are therefore advisable.

Confirming adequate balloon occlusion

Complete antral and ostial cryolesions require circumferential balloon–tissue contact and can be accomplished only by seamless balloon occlusion with pulmonary venous flow coming to a complete stop. Any leakage will increase local blood flow velocity and create turbulent flow similar to the mechanisms at the site of a vascular stenosis. This results in diminished or abolished freezing at some portion of the vein circumference and thereby leads to incomplete or only temporary isolation of the vein. Ascertaining balloon occlusion angiographically is fraught with two pitfalls: (1) after the initial low-pressure inflation of the balloon, it changes its shape and size when full refrigerant flow is delivered. This can make the balloon slide backward or tilt, creating new leaks that cannot be detected because the lumen is now beginning to freeze. (2) Respiratory-induced motion of the cardiac base or the effect of phrenic nerve stimulation can move the balloon intermittently and create leaks that also go undetected during the freezing process.

At our center, we therefore opted to (1) first ascertain proper balloon position with the balloon inflated at a low pressure, and then (2) perform a second injection with diluted contrast agent after commencing the freezing process. Verifying balloon position in the modified (i.e., the final) balloon configuration is an advance because it provides the opportunity to increase the balloon–tissue contact, guaranteeing complete occlusion. This is obviously feasible only during the first minute of the freezing process until a flow of approximately 45 sccm is reached and prior to the injection channel freezing

shut. In 600 patients, we did not observe any problems related to the channel becoming inaccessible for flushing with saline or due to the mixture of blood and contrast agent freezing. These issues are of a temporary nature because rewarming causes rapid thawing.

This method has the added advantage of permitting balloon size and configuration adjustments aimed to prevent balloon slippage into the vein in cases where the pulmonary vein antrum can be stretched beyond the nominal balloon diameter. Additionally, an undersized balloon can be pulled back at the time of the first angiogram, so that some refluxing contrast agent helps depict the true pulmonary vein ostium. One can also wait for the balloon to expand when the freezing process starts in order to advance the now-stiffened balloon to the antrum (Figure 5.5). This technique precludes inadvertent balloon slippage into the pulmonary vein and facilitates correct antral and ostial placement of the freezing balloon. Leaks can be conclusively detected at an early time.

Similar to the pulmonary wedge pressure tracing with a Swan–Ganz catheter depicting a pulmonary venous pressure curve, the fluid column in the catheter transmits a pulmonary arterial pressure curve when the pulmonary vein is completely occluded.

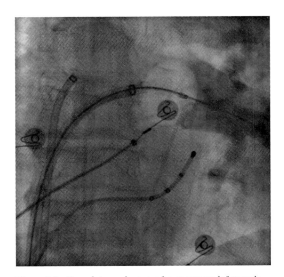

Figure 5.5. Complete occlusion of a common left trunk by cryoballoon. The balloon was initially inflated at the ostium with no occlusion. At the start of freezing, the balloon was advanced towards the ostium and occlusion was confirmed with dye of freeze.

This pressure tracing is easily distinguishable from the pulmonary venous pressure curve and can verify the degree of occlusion until the fluid column begins to freeze.[6]

A superior method to check for leaks during the initial freezing phase and during the actual freezing process is transesophageal echocardiography (TEE) monitoring, which can also be accomplished when the lumen is frozen shut. TEE facilitates correction and closure of discovered leaks by monitoring subsequent balloon adjustments, a major advantage of this method. While under just analgo-sedation, patients cannot be expected to tolerate TEE for the entire duration of the procedure. The requirement for general anesthesia is a shortcoming of TEE monitoring.[7]

Intracardiac echocardiography (ICE) represents a particularly elegant method. Not only is it capable of guiding the septal puncture, but also it helps detect complications. All pulmonary veins can be visualized. The spatial relationship between balloon and vein antrum can be visualized. Detecting leaks and monitoring corrective measures are equally straightforward. ICE also helps the operator decide when to abort because of incomplete occlusion. Leaks can be clearly distinguished from the normal flow pattern of the adjacent pulmonary vein. The degree of occlusion depicted by ICE correlates very well with the long-term success of vein isolation.[8] Disadvantages of this method include additional expenditures, for which health insurance providers in some countries do not provide reimbursement, and the need for inserting an additional large-bore femoral venous sheath.

Impact of pulmonary vein anatomy

Anatomical variations of the pulmonary veins are frequent. In 8–10% of cases, there is a common ostium or a common trunk on the left side. Both these variations are challenging if the opening is wider than 28 mm, especially when the ostium can be stretched even further. With currently available balloons, a sequential approach to isolation is required in such cases.

Right-sided common trunks are rarely encountered. A right middle lobe vein is not unusual, but an isolated middle lobe vein orifice is uncommon because the middle lobe vein tends to drain into the ostium or antrum of the right superior or inferior pulmonary vein, making the entire ostium accessible for isolation with the same freeze.

Accessory veins draining into the atrial roof are more unusual and will often remain undetected until patients undergo preprocedural imaging studies. Isolation of these small ostia is challenging. The same holds true for a right middle lobe vein with a separate atrial ostium, particularly when a large balloon is used.

It is very unusual to encounter three left pulmonary veins.

The shape of the pulmonary vein ostia is highly variable. It is well known that the ostia are not actually round, but more oval and occasionally slit-like.[9] The right upper vein is often funnel shaped, whereas the left upper vein ostium tends to have a more longish cylindrical shape. On the septal side, the right lower vein divides very quickly into side branches. The left lower vein drains posteriorly and is more frequently cylindrical but short or tapers toward its conical ostium. This makes isolation procedures more difficult because the balloon does not have much support on the surrounding flat atrial wall: riding on just the rim of the vein, the balloon is mostly surrounded by flowing blood.

A circumferential sleeve of contractile muscle tissue often encircles the left upper vein, a finding more uncommon at the right upper vein. Atrial contraction will frequently lead to underestimation of vein diameters unless electrocardiogram (ECG)-triggered dynamic imaging is used.

Depending on their filling state, left atrial pressure, and cardiac rhythm, pulmonary veins can be quite distensible so that their diameter is underestimated, especially at the antral level. Large studies (e.g., a study on more than 600 patients treated at our center) have revealed that the upper veins are significantly larger than the lower veins. Isolation procedures in rigid and maximally distended veins are particularly challenging because large balloons cannot adapt to these ostia.

The myocardial sleeves in the vicinity of the carina separating ipsilateral veins are often thicker than at the remainder of the venous circumference. Sleeve length is also variable: the left upper sleeve is the longest one, and the right upper and right lower myocardial sleeves are the shortest ones. After isolation, it is therefore crucial to pay particular attention to residual electrical potentials in these veins. Especially on the left, the upper and lower veins can have muscular bridges leading to the so-called crosstalk phenomenon between veins: upper vein isolation appears to fail until the carinal aspect of the lower vein has been isolated. The frequency of crosstalk tends to be overestimated, however, because asymmetric balloon positions can easily result in inadequate cooling of the inferior hemicircumference of the veins in proximity to the balloon shaft.

Impact of balloon characteristics

The refrigerant enters through high-velocity injectors. Equatorial distribution toward the four quadrants of the inner balloon is most important. Although the cycle flow $\rightarrow$ vaporization $\rightarrow$ vacuum $\rightarrow$ backflow favors ice formation at the impact sites of the jets, cooling is relatively uniform, even toward the balloon tip. The most intense ice formation occurs along an equatorial band; cooling is least at the balloon tip in the vicinity of the shaft. In this region, it fails to elicit a transmural lesion.

With the balloon optimally centered and pulmonary venous flow fully arrested, one can expect a lesion of optimal width at the balloon–wall contact area. Such a lesion will also have the proper transmural depth (Figure 5.6).

If the balloon is asymmetrically positioned at the vein ostium – this occurs frequently when isolating the long cylinder-shaped left upper vein or when the balloon is supported from the atrial roof and pointed toward the often small lower veins (Figure 5.6) – gaps will form close to the shaft, typically inferiorly. This explains the location of most gaps reported in the literature.

By occluding small-caliber and early branching veins with a large balloon near the ostium, one will often create lesions that are too narrow and end up being unreliable. Especially small lower veins with a conical taper toward the ostium are often not amenable to reliable occlusion and isolation with a large balloon because only the warmer area near the catheter shaft is in nearly circumferential contact with ostial tissue (Figure 5.7).

Until more refined cryoballoons became available, our individualized approach to anatomical variations proved successful. Long-term follow-ups demonstrated that the single big-balloon strategy was associated with a higher recurrence rate than the double big- and small-balloon strategy.[10]

The fact that the balloon becomes harder and nonpliable when N_2O is instilled is a shortcoming of today's balloon technology. Increased balloon rigidity can lead to positional changes, leaks, and loss of optimal occlusion. Accidental inflation inside a vein is associated with the risk of a percutaneous transluminal angioplasty (PTA)-like effect.

Imaging

Preprocedural magnetic resonance imaging (MRI) of the left atrium and pulmonary veins is advisable

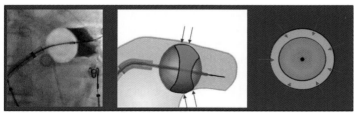

Optimal Contact Area of Coldest Balloon Parts

Asymmetric Occlusion Creates Inferior Gaps

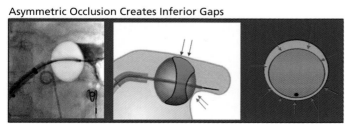

Figure 5.6. Top: Optimal contact area of coldest balloon parts; bottom: asymmetric occlusion creates inferior gaps. (Figure created by N. Bogunovic.)

Large Balloon Occludes Small Vein: Slim Lesion Only

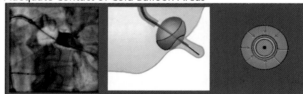

Mismatch of Small Veln With Flat Left Atrial Balloon:
No Adequate Contact of Cold Balloon Areas

Figure 5.7. Top: Large balloon occludes small vein; slim lesion only. Bottom: Mismatch of small vein with flat left atrial wall and large balloon: no adequate contact of cold balloon areas. (Figure created by N. Bogunovic.)

because it can depict large common trunks and isolated accessory veins prior to isolation.

Selective pulmonary vein angiography either through the transseptal sheath or through an angiography catheter (e.g., an NIH 6F catheter) has become a standard part of the procedure. Angiography can supplement still radiographs that depict the anatomic landmarks.

Another option is angiography of the entire left atrium and the pulmonary veins under adenosine-induced asystole or during rapid right ventricular pacing. This method's shortcomings include overestimation of size and filling, because normal left atrial activity is associated with muscular contraction of the atrium and the proximal pulmonary vein segments.

Dyna computed tomography (CT) of the left atrium and the pulmonary veins is reconstructed from rotational angiography images. Superimposition of the current fluoroscopic view with a three-dimensional representation automatically adjusted for the current fluoroscopic projection provides a particularly elegant aid for navigation.

Intraprocedural ICE imaging provides superior definition of the vein antrum, the common antra, and the relationship between balloon and antrum, and permits recognition of leaks and proper occlusion. This method may also be helpful for depicting how close the inferior vein is to the esophagus.

Using pulmonary vein morphology and size information derived from MRI sequences that were obtained without ECG gating while the underlying cardiac rhythm differed from that at the time of the intervention (e.g., atrial fibrillation vs. sinus rhythm) does not make sense. Different filling states and different phases of pulmonary vein contraction or relaxation (isolation and reconnection can contribute to this issue) can lead to a false positive diagnosis of pulmonary vein stenosis or enlargement after the intervention.

Special isolation techniques

Left upper pulmonary vein

Most often, the left upper pulmonary vein is the vein with the most complex anatomy. Superiorly, the vein circumference merges directly with the thickest section of the muscle on the atrial roof. A part of the ganglionated plexus is located proximal to the antrum. A guidewire touching this region can elicit a vagal response including sinus arrest as well as complete AV block, a phenomenon even more frequent with the Achieve catheter. Another issue is the proximity of the left main bronchus, which can be affected when ice forms. An urge to cough is often evoked during the thawing phase and/or after thawing. An additional factor is the lumen of the left atrial appendage, which is connected via an anteriorly bordering ridge of variable width. The left superior vein is often long and cylindrical, so that the relationship between balloon and antrum does not change when either the Achieve catheter or the guidewire is advanced into one of the various side branches. The length of the sleeve makes the left upper pulmonary vein the most suitable vein for pulmonary vein signal monitoring during the freezing phase. If the pulmonary vein potentials do not disappear, one has to rule out either remote potentials from the left atrial appendage (LAA) or crosstalk between the inferior segment of the vein wall and the left inferior vein. LAA remote potentials can be recognized by LAA stimulation. If crosstalk is suspected, one should commence with lower vein isolation after the second freeze. In cases of large vein antra, it is advisable to rotate the catheter anteriorly after isolation in order to check for a connection with the LAA. If the area of the ridge cannot be isolated, one can aim to perform transmural ablation of the ridge by carefully positioning the balloon in the proximal LAA and by rotating it clockwise prior to the freezing cycle. If the balloon occludes the LAA completely, the freeze should be terminated when the Achieve signals disappear in order to avoid permanent complete isolation of the LAA (Figure 5.8; and see Video Clip 5.3)

A common trunk or a common ostium with a diameter of more than 28–30 mm requires sequential ablation beginning at the posterior and superior aspect, then advancing to the superior and anterior portion before completing ostial isolation by pro-ceeding to the infero-posterior and infero-anterior regions. Wide leaks at the unsupported side of the balloon have to be accepted. Complete isolation will often require 5–6 freezes.

Left lower pulmonary vein

The left lower pulmonary vein is often smaller. It is essential to center the balloon over the vein either inferiorly or horizontally with a juxtaposed sheath. The guide should be maximally deflected if the sheath and the balloon deviate superiorly. Deflection of the guide forces the balloon from a superior location inferiorly against the vein antrum. This so-called hockey stick technique is most successful when the Achieve catheter is directly advanced into the lower side branch after pushing the balloon against the antrum. The guide is then used as a rail for guiding the balloon. If a leak is observed at the lower aspect of the vein circumference, it can be closed by traction on the sheath, which moves the balloon caudally (the so-called pull-down technique).

In that situation, the duration of freezing may have to be extended in order to create complete lesions in these areas. The pull-down technique described here is reliable. Monitoring shows that time to isolation is often as short as 10–20 sec. If the pull-down maneuver is effective, the temperature curve drops abruptly by 5–10 °C.[11]

Right upper pulmonary vein

As the right upper pulmonary vein is more often funnel shaped than the other veins, the balloon is prone to slip too far into the vein. The risk of phrenic nerve palsy makes it advisable to select the largest balloon available. The best backup for balloon alignment and balloon force is achieved by advancing the Achieve catheter far into the upper main branch. Since the vein merges directly with the left atrial roof, the balloon axis can be displaced horizontally. The balloon will still be in satisfactory contact with the superior edge of the vein, but there will be an inferior leak, the size of which increases periodically during respiration or under phrenic nerve stimulation. In this case, the pull-down technique should be used. A better alternative is repositioning of the Achieve catheter into the side branch that enters caudally, a technique that permits inferior tilting of the balloon while completely occluding the superior aspect of the antrum at the same

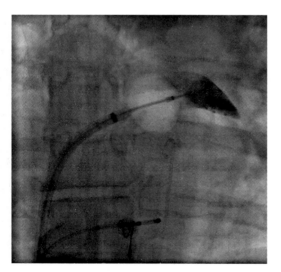

Figure 5.8. Freezing of the left atrial appendage in order to ablate the otherwise intractable ridge.

time. Rigorous phrenic nerve monitoring by direct proximal nerve stimulation from the superior vena cava is mandatory. Since the right-sided myocardial sleeves are not that long, vein potential monitoring is often impossible. After the freezes, the proximal vein has to be thoroughly checked for potentials.

Right lower pulmonary vein

Because the right inferior pulmonary vein is so close to the septal puncture site, it is the most difficult vein to ablate. This applies to all ablation techniques. The actual distance between vein and puncture site determines if the vein can be reached directly by clockwise rotation or if one has to resort to a loop technique. If the transseptal puncture site is not too far posterior, the ostium is accessible even if the atrium is small. At our center, we first retract the balloon well into the Flexcath sheath. The Achieve catheter spiral remains directly in front of the sheath. The sheath is maximally deflected and rotated clockwise toward the ostium of the inferior vein. Pulmonary vein spikes from the rather short sleeves are immediately detectable. The Achieve catheter can be advanced far into the lower side branch caudally when the sheath is deflected. It acts as a rail, guiding the balloon catheter until the entire balloon can unfold between the ostium and the tip of the sheath. Finally, the Achieve catheter valve at the balloon catheter handle is closed, so that the sheath cannot be forced back during balloon inflation.

By trapping the balloon as described, the antrum can be completely covered when the balloon is inflated. A size mismatch between balloon and the often smallish vein leads to an inferior leak that can be closed by the pull-down technique or by using the push-up technique after freezing the lower antrum first. If the anatomy is challenging, the loop technique can be applied, either by forming a large loop or by supporting the sheath at the left-sided veins. Another option is the hockey stick technique, which involves pushing balloon and sheath cranially.[11,12]

Loop techniques are more challenging with the current type of sheaths, which should not only allow more deflection but also come equipped with a longer tip with a dorsal orientation and be controlled by an asymmetrically attached pull-wire.

Anatomically, the right lower vein is often smaller and quickly divides into two or three branches. Isolation is technically straightforward when the ostium points horizontally or cranially. If the ostium is directed toward the left atrial floor, isolation is challenging.

During more than 700 cryoballoon ablation procedures at our center, we did not see a single case of phrenic nerve paralysis due to ablation of the right inferior pulmonary vein. Single cases have been reported in the literature, however. Large or dominant (in relation to the right upper pulmonary vein) right lower veins tend to be associated with this complication. In both situations, one should use phrenic nerve stimulation as described for the right upper pulmonary vein.

Confirming isolation

Until October 2010, we used 10- or 20-electrode Lasso catheters in some cases to confirm the presence of pulmonary vein spikes before isolation and to verify the absence of spikes thereafter. Placing two transseptal sheaths, we could verify isolation of all treated veins immediately after each freeze and after a waiting period. This technique is also capable of elegantly demonstrating the so-called crosstalk between left-sided veins. A Lasso catheter with an adjustable loop diameter is advantageous because it can monitor the entire antral circumference, even in large veins, and can detect any residual signals. We initially confirmed entrance block by coronary sinus stimulation for the left-sided veins and by right atrial stimulation for the right-sided veins. If isolation was in doubt (and for study purposes), we looked for an exit block by performing bipolar stimulation with a Lasso catheter. With only a single septal sheath, all veins were subsequently isolated with an average number of two freezes. The balloon catheter was then replaced by the Lasso catheter. Any residual conduction necessitated yet another change of catheters. At our center, we therefore decided to always use three freezes for the left upper pulmonary vein. There was no evidence of a dose–response relationship. Exchanging catheters might increase the risk of thromboembolic events and air embolism.

For redo procedures, it seems advisable to check all veins with the Lasso catheter first right after transseptal puncture. The results will then provide the basis for planning the reisolation strategy.

The newly developed Achieve catheter with eight electrodes combines a guidewire property with very

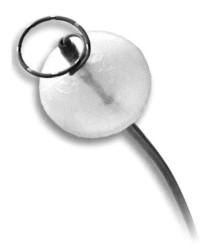

Figure 5.9. Achieve catheter. (Reproduced with permission of Medtronic, Inc.)

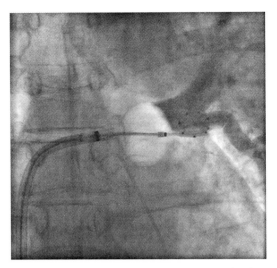

Figure 5.10. Combination of proven occlusion and withdrawal of Achieve catheter.

good backup and a spiral catheter that is insertable through the inner lumen for detecting pulmonary vein signals, permitting one to confirm isolation without having to change catheters (Figure 5.9). Other than with the Lasso catheter, which needs the best possible circumferential apposition to the wall, lack of the cascade of pulmonary vein spikes can be demonstrated with the Achieve catheter, even when the apposition is incomplete, and is indicative of an entrance block.

If there is any doubt, the Achieve catheter as well as the Lasso catheter can be used to check for an exit block.

As the Achieve catheter doubles as a guidewire, it will have to be advanced into small side branches. Therefore, it is advisable to use the 20 mm version for large veins. If all veins are smaller, the 15 mm version will be easier to manipulate. Using the smaller Achieve diameter for isolation testing of large veins does not have any shortcomings.

In cases of a common ostium, a common trunk, or a large left upper vein, one should look for residual signals at the ridge anteriorly.

The Achieve catheter guarantees a stable balloon position. A standard intervention can therefore be completed without having to change over to a guidewire. At our Center, the introduction of the Achieve catheter helped us decrease the procedure time to less than 2 h and the fluoroscopy time to less than 20 min.

Monitoring pulmonary vein signals

The real progress brought by the Achieve catheter is the ability to monitor pulmonary vein signals during cryoisolation. For monitoring, the Achieve catheter needs to be pulled back to the level of the catheter tip after balloon placement, possibly as late as during the first minute of freezing while contrast agent is being injected (Figure 5.10; and see Video Clip 5.4). Unless the muscle sleeves are long enough and the long catheter tip does not reach too far into the vein, vein spikes can be immediately detected and distinguished from left atrial potentials. In cases of complete occlusion, the spikes become progressively delayed before 2:1 conduction develops and before the spikes eventually disappear completely. A particularly clear-cut sign of isolation is a dissociated rhythm in the vein but no conduction, for example atrial fibrillation or even pulmonary vein tachycardia restricted to the isolated vein, but sinus rhythm on the surface ECG (Figures 5.11, 5.12, and 5.13).

Due to the rather long balloon tip and relatively short myocardial sleeves, especially on the right side, monitoring can currently catch only 50–60% of vein signals. Nevertheless, being able to detect whether vein isolation was successful after each freeze is a clear advantage, particularly if the tissue is quickly recovering or if isolation failed. If a vein with an inferior leak can be successfully monitored,

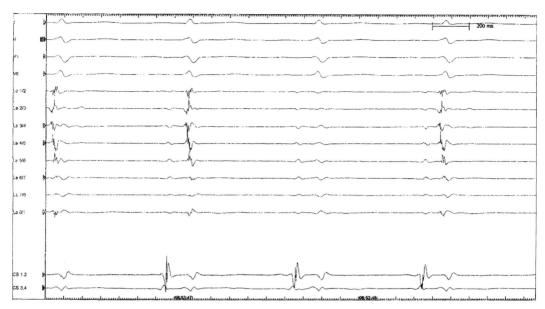

Figure 5.11. 2:1 conduction of myocardial sleeve during isolation.

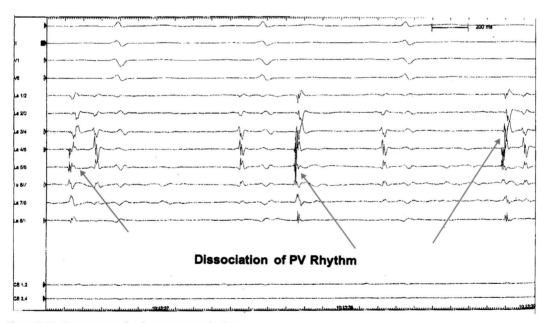

Figure 5.12. Dissociation of pulmonary vein rhythm.

one can directly observe if the pull-down maneuver eliminates the spikes and can prolong the freezing time accordingly.

Various authors who used the Achieve catheter's predecessor (i.e., the Promap catheter) have reported that veins with a short time to isolation remained permanently isolated. Therefore, a second freeze can be viewed as a "bonus freeze" for making the lesion more homogeneous. Still, the region of overlap between short and long times to isolation clearly necessitates a waiting period, confirmation, and bonus freezes.[13–15]

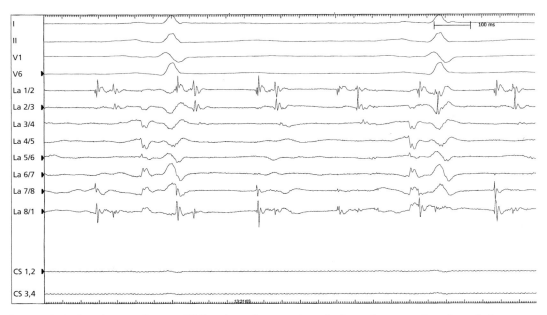

Figure 5.13. Surface electrocardiogram (ECG) with simultaneous sinus rhythm; pulmonary vein tachycardia in an isolated large left common ostium.

Benefits of the Achieve Catheter

- Time to isolation monitoring
- Detection of early reconduction
- Demonstrating isolation and conduction after every freeze
- Reduction of freezing time, procedure duration, and fluoroscopy time
- Definition of bonus impulses
- Avoiding multiple catheter changes over one large sheath

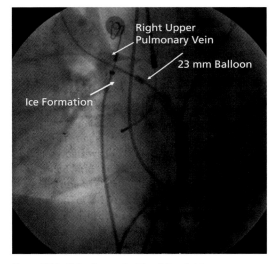

Figure 5.14. Polar icecap inside of the right upper pulmonary vein properly occluded by a 23 mm balloon.

Risk of phrenic nerve palsy

Due to the anatomic proximity between the right phrenic nerve and the superior vena cava (SVC), the superior portion of the right atrium, and especially the ostium of the right superior pulmonary vein, all types of catheter ablation for atrial fibrillation are associated with the risk of right phrenic nerve paralysis. Worldwide, the incidence of permanent phrenic nerve paralysis is 0.17%. While wide antral ablation with RF energy prevents right phrenic

nerve injury, the cryoballoon is forced against the ostium of the right upper and right lower pulmonary vein. Especially small-diameter balloons lead to rapid cooling and significant ice formation near the antrum, particularly at the ostium, and also in the vein lumen (Figure 5.14; and see Video Clip

5.5). At the ostium of the right upper and – provided it is large – the right lower pulmonary veins, the risk of phrenic nerve palsy increases the deeper the balloon is positioned and frozen. In the initial three-center study, the reported incidence of phrenic nerve damage was 7.5%. Most of these complication occurred with 23 mm balloons. In this early period, there was a learning process in the technique of checking diaphragmatic motion radiographically in intervals of 30–60 s toward phrenic nerve stimulation from the superior vena cava above the occluded pulmonary vein.[16]

In small series, rates of phrenic nerve paralysis were reported to be in the range of 4.7–14%. In larger series, the incidence decreased to 3%.[11,12,16–19] In a population of more than 600 patients treated at our center, the incidence was 2%. In 10 of these, a 23 mm balloon was used; in two, a 28 mm balloon. Among the most recent 420 patients, the incidence was only 0.7% – due to consistent phrenic nerve stimulation and monitoring. All cases of phrenic nerve palsy were temporary, and nerve function recovered completely by one year or earlier, occasionally as early as after 3–6 months. Few transient nerve paralyses with recovery after several minutes were observed in 50% with the small balloon and 50% with the large one.

Anomalous courses of the phrenic nerve in the vicinity of the ostium of the right lower pulmonary vein have been described, as well as cases of temporary paralysis after isolation of a very large right lower pulmonary vein. These observations are not congruent with the results of large studies. Antral occlusion offers the best protection against phrenic nerve injury, and so does continuous monitoring of diaphragmatic contraction under phrenic nerve stimulation.

A multi-electrode catheter advanced from the femoral vein into the superior vena cava provides the most reliable stimulation. Using the upside-down technique, the catheter is opened toward the dorsolateral wall of the SVC (Figure 5.15; and see Video Clip 5.6). For improved capture, a wide electrical field is created by bipolar stimulation between the distal and the third electrode.

With increasing experience, examiners will develop an awareness for progressively diminishing excursion of the right hemidiaphragm, which indicates that transient phrenic nerve palsy is turning into persistent palsy. The excursion of the dia-

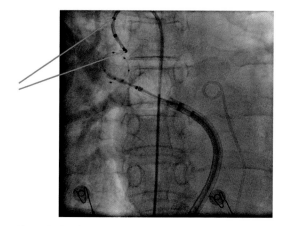

Figure 5.15. Phrenic nerve pacing (superior vena cava): upside-down technique of phrenic nerve pacing. Optimal occlusion and alignment of the right upper pulmonary vein with a 28 mm balloon.

phragm can be felt through the abdominal wall, but the palpatory findings cannot be quantitated easily. Even minimal displacement of the stimulation catheter changes the amplitude of excursion. The latter is also modulated by the respiratory cycle. The crucial time for thawing can therefore be missed. If general anesthesia is used, the difference between diaphragmatic contraction due to stimulation and spontaneous excursion not inducible by inspiration can go unnoticed. In these cases, phrenic nerve palsy will not be detected until a chest X-ray is taken in full inspiration.

The recently reported method of recording the electrical summation potentials originating from the right hemidiaphragm is particularly helpful for detecting incipient phrenic nerve damage. Monitoring is easily accomplished by attaching one of the ECG limb lead I electrodes to the xiphoid process and the other to the skin directly below the middle of the right costal margin.[20] With increased amplification, the tracing will then depict the stimulation spike, immediately followed by the electrical summation potential of the diaphragm. The signal amplitude dropping to 60% indicates incipient phrenic nerve paralysis (Figure 5.16a and 5.16b). Freezing can then be terminated on time. Watching hepatic excursion by ICE is another semiquantitative method. For this, the ICE catheter is pulled back

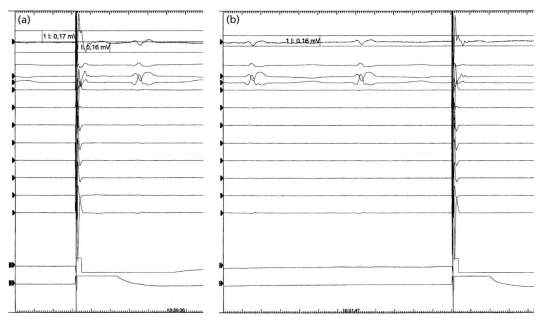

Figure 5.16. Reduction of amplitude. (a) Begin of freeze of the right upper pulmonary vein: large diaphragm signal behind the spike. (b) Loss of 50% amplitude of diaphragm signal with transient loss of spontaneous diaphragm innervation.

into the inferior vena cava (personal communication from Dr. Marcin Kowalski, Staten Island, NY).

Frequently asked questions

How should one respond to transient phrenic nerve paralysis after 2–4 min of freezing with the 28 mm balloon?

If vein isolation is successful at that time, one does not have to continue. Keep in mind, though, that a redo procedure may be required in the future. If the vein has not been isolated, one can repeat the freeze, but it should be kept shorter than the aborted freezing time before so that no transient phrenic nerve damage occurs. The final alternative is the Lasso-guided touch-up technique with a cryoablation or RF single-tip catheter.

Phrenic nerve pacing fails from the superior vena cava. What are the options?

Alternative sites are the confluence of the subclavian vein with the superior vena cava and the azygos vein. Both sites offer good phrenic nerve capture.

> **Phrenic nerve notes**
>
> • In experienced hands, the risk of phrenic nerve palsy can be lower than 1%.
> • Phrenic nerve stimulation from the superior vena cava and electrical monitoring of the right hemidiaphragm are essential.
> • In cases of large right lower pulmonary veins, such monitoring will also increase safety.

Other adverse events

Stroke and transient ischemic attack

Theoretically, ablation with cryoenergy should be the least thrombogenic approach. Other than RF energy, cryoenergy does not disrupt the intima. This is in line with transcranial Doppler studies detecting lower numbers of microemboli. Current publications confirm a trend toward a lower incidence of clinically silent emboli with cryoablation when compared to cooled RF ablation. Compared to noncooled dual uni- and bipolar ablation systems, cooled RF and cryoablation are associated with a highly significantly lower incidence of thromboembolism.[21–24]

In addition to thromboembolism, suction and valve effects can lead to air embolism, primarily as a consequence of catheters being advanced or pulled back inside a large sheath and due to manipulation of the Achieve catheter and injection of contrast agent through the same lumen. Cerebral air emboli can remain clinically silent or become symptomatic; coronary air emboli may lead to temporary myocardial ischemia with ST elevation. The ischemia is most often inferior because with the patient supine, the right coronary artery takes off from the highest point of the aortic root where air is most likely to collect. For treatment, it is usually sufficient to just sedate the patient, administer a parasympatholytic agent, and wait for a couple of minutes for the ST elevation to regress. Large amounts of air collecting in the left atrial appendage can be identified on (native) fluoroscopy and must be removed by catheter suction.

In our large cohort, the incidence of strokes or TIAs was fortunately only 0.3% (two patients). Both patients recovered completely.

Pulmonary vein stenosis

Pulmonary vein stenosis is a known and feared complication of RF ablation, especially of segmental ablation. After most centers adopted wide atrial encircling of the pulmonary veins, the incidence of pulmonary vein stenosis decreased to 1.3% worldwide. Because cryoenergy preserves the extracellular matrix and the intima, cryoablation is not expected to be associated with pulmonary vein stenosis. Experienced centers report a very low incidence of pulmonary vein stenosis. At our center, we have performed more than 600 cryoballoon procedures after we had already gained experience with more than 200 procedures completed with the curvilinear cryoablation catheter. On systematic MRI follow-up examinations of our entire population over a period of up to 2 years after ablation, only two cases of pulmonary vein stenosis were detected. One of these occurred in a location remote and distal to the balloon site, and the other after a redo ablation procedure with RF energy.[25–27]

Pulmonary vein stenoses were reported in more recent publications, however (e.g., in the Sustained Treatment of Paroxysmal Atrial Fibrillation [STOP AF] trial and in case reports). The reported cases were probably the result of less experience as illustrated by some of the balloon positions documented in these publications, including flat profiles and balloons positioned inside pulmonary veins. Such factors can explain a PTA-like effect with subsequent damage to the vein wall due to the inflation pressure and the pressure increase during ice formation.

To avoid this complication, the cryoballoon cannot be expanded within the lumen of a vein, nor should full refrigerant flow commence when the balloon is in that position. Either could damage the vein wall and may even lead to vein rupture, a complication that has been reported once.

Left atrial esophageal fistula

Experimental and clinical studies have shown that the ice forming at the cryoballoon can extend to the epicardial surface of the left atrium and beyond. Impressive images of esophageal constriction and spasm have been recorded.[28,29] Especially the inferior veins, which enter the left atrium from posterior, are in close proximity to the esophagus if the latter is not directly centered behind the left atrium. Esophageal temperatures below 0 °C have been recorded experimentally and clinically, and in 17% were correlated with esophageal ulcerations detected by endoscopy on the day after ablation.[30] Such changes were not observed with 28 mm balloons.[31]

Atrial-esophageal fistulas are most often fatal. Although the detailed etiology is not always completely understood, the following pathophysiological mechanisms are thought to contribute: thermal ablation of the blood supply of the esophagus, thermal injury to the esophageal wall, and damage to the parasympathetic plexus and nerves with subsequent reflux.[32] It remains to be seen if the prophylactic administration of proton pump inhibitors, which are known to improve ulcer healing, can also prevent fistulas. Both cryoenergy and RF energy can cause thermal injury. Two fatal fistulas were recently observed, one in Germany and one in the United States. According to personal communications, both were probably due to very distal balloon positions or very low temperatures in the inferior veins.[33]

Dysphagia after the ablation procedure, which has been reported, may be a warning of collateral damage extending beyond the left atrial wall.[17]

Therefore, the most important caveat for preventing left atrial esophageal fistulas is to ablate the antrum and to stay well away from the inferior vein lumen.

Cough and hemoptysis

Balloon placement and manipulation of the guidewire or Achieve catheter are frequently accompanied by an urge to cough. Fluoroscopically, one can easily appreciate the close proximity between the left upper pulmonary vein and left main bronchus and notice compression of the bronchus when ice forms. These observations and a published case of an endobronchial erosion confirm the impact of the procedure on the bronchus.[34]

Hemoptysis was reported in initial animal experiments and in the early clinical studies on the cryoballoon. Hemoptysis is usually not caused by guidewire injury, but by lung tissue being affected. This cannot always be prevented, unless the balloon is too deep within the vein. CT scans in patients with hemoptysis consistently show a pulmonary vein thickened to the adventitia and surrounded by hematoma and edema (Figure 5.17; and see Video Clips 5.7 and 5.8). These alterations heal without

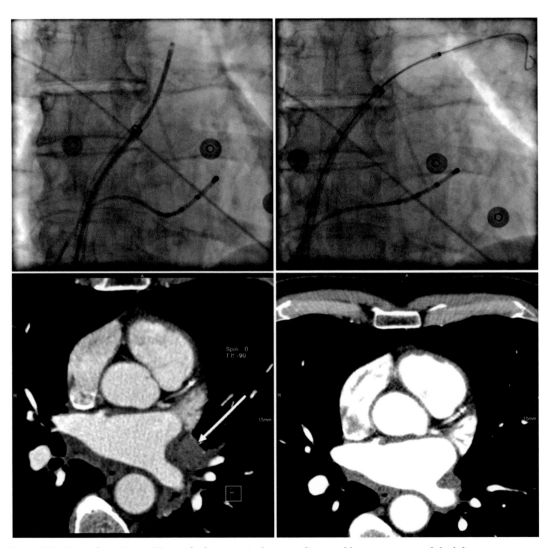

Figure 5.17. Frozen lung tissue: CT scan for hemoptysis showing edema and hematoma around the left upper pulmonary vein and between the left ipsilateral veins. Complete reduction after 4 weeks.

deleterious effects; hemoptysis improves after 2–4 days, and does not lead to infectious complications. Nevertheless, too deep a balloon position should always be avoided. Other than after RF ablation, no fistulas between the left atrium or the pulmonary vein and the bronchial system have been reported.

Headaches

All patients report headaches at various locations. This phenomenon can be explained by nerve connections with the trigeminal nerve branches supplying the face. Especially when freezing of a vein commences, pain can be extremely intense, but will diminish the longer the freeze lasts. Liberal administration of analgesics is recommended. Intense intrathoracic pain during inferior vein isolation is a warning sign for the vein being overextended and for too deep a balloon position. If this occurs during freezes in the vicinity of the right upper vein, it can be a warning sign for incipient phrenic nerve palsy.

Pericardial effusion and pericardial tamponade

Pericardial tamponade is not specific for ablation with cryoenergy, because it is always caused by technical errors with transseptal puncture or catheter manipulation (e.g., maneuvering of the coronary sinus or stimulation catheter in the right atrium or the superior vena cava, or unprotected manipulation of the sheath). Physicians performing ablation procedures have to be proficient in pericardial aspiration to be able to treat pericardial tamponade.

Late tamponade is a dreaded complication reported after RF ablation.[35] This entity has not been observed after cryoablation. Also, pericardial effusion accompanying cryoballoon therapy has not been reported by experienced centers.

Left atrial flutter and left atrial macro-reentrant tachycardias

Point-by-point ablation and pulmonary vein encircling with RF energy have doubled the worldwide incidence of iatrogenic left atrial tachycardias.[35] By comparison, this type of arrhythmia is extremely rare after cryoballoon ablation. Inhomogeneous lesion formation and lesions that do not reach the full transmural thickness in cases of a very thick antral muscle layer would be the only real explanation for such an arrhythmia. Perimitral flutter can

also occur and is obviously not dependent on the type of energy used for ablation.

> **Avoiding adverse events, complications, and unreliable lesions**
>
> • A large balloon is mandatory for antral isolation in large veins and common trunks.
> • Small veins below 18 mm diameter show a small antrum with effective overlap due to a small balloon.
> • Using a small balloon in all veins results in just ostial isolation and jeopardizes lung tissue, the esophagus, and the pulmonary vein walls (PTA-like effect).
> • The equatorial freezing profile of today's balloons and asymmetric cooling create unreliable lesions (hockey stick technique).

Anticoagulation

At our center, patients on phenprocoumon did not interrupt this drug regimen when undergoing ablation. This approach has been used since the cryoballoon became available and for cryoablation with the single-tip catheter or with the self-expanding curvilinear spiral catheter. We did not observe an increased rate of complications in procedures requiring single or dual transseptal punctures if the INR was in the range of 2.0 to 3.0.

Simultaneously with transseptal puncture, we administer either a heparin bolus of 100 units per kg of body weight or a single dose of 10 000 units. During the subsequent course, the ACT is checked in half-hour intervals. Additional boluses are given to maintain an ACT greater than 300–350 s. The heparin effect is not reversed at the end of the procedure. Anticoagulation is continued for 6 weeks to 3 months in patients with a $CHADS_2DS_2$–VASc Score of 0 or 1. In accordance with current guidelines, patients with a higher score are kept on phenprocoumon beyond this period. More recent oral anticoagulants were used only in individual cases. One needs to be aware of the risk–benefit ratio and the lack of antagonists for some of these types of medications.

Results of cryoballoon ablation

The number of randomized follow-up studies on the results of cryoballoon ablation is limited. As early as 2008, the German three-center trial demonstrated that at a mean follow-up period of 1 year, freedom from atrial fibrillation off drugs was 74% in patients with paroxysmal atrial fibrillation and only 42% in patients with persistent atrial fibrillation. When using balloons, only 97% of the pulmonary veins could be isolated. A second nonrandomized study comparing cryoablation with RF ablation revealed similar results. Freedom from atrial fibrillation after 12 months was 77% in patients with paroxysmal versus 48% in patients with persistent atrial fibrillation. The interventional techniques were not fully comparable. Using balloons only, 83% of the pulmonary veins could be isolated.[16,36]

Meta-analyses revealed that both the acute per vein and the per patient success rates were 98%. The 1-year success rate in patients with paroxysmal atrial fibrillation was 72% when events during the blanking period were disregarded and 60% counting all events, and 45% in patients with persistent atrial fibrillation.[37]

So far, long-term data with follow-up periods extending over several years are available only as single-center reports or abstracts. A paper with our 1- to 6-year follow-up data has recently been published[38] and confirms that the outcome remains very stable over time.

Outlook and future development

So far, the literature has demonstrated that for treating paroxysmal atrial fibrillation, the results of cryoballoon ablation are not inferior to the results of RF ablation. As of now, the required learning curve, the rather straightforward intervention, and a low risk of side effects appear to favor balloon ablation.

Transmural freezing of the complete surface of the pulmonary vein antrum can possibly better fulfill the dream of persistent pulmonary vein isolation by a low-risk procedure as first-line therapy than point-to-point RF ablation. One may even envision hybrid procedures for the management of advanced atrial disease and successful extension of this technology to the ablation of rotors.

Desirable advancements in balloon system design include a higher ratio of cooling power to balloon size as well as more homogeneous cooling of the balloon surface, which would facilitate the ablation of crosstalk, inferior reconduction, and gaps. Small balloon diameters would then be required only to isolate veins that have a special anatomy. In fact, a larger balloon will be needed to replace the make-shift sequential technique currently used for ablating common ostia and trunks. Only time will tell if the size and durability of cryolesions will justify again extending the indication to the large group of patients with heart failure and persistent atrial fibrillation.

If permanent pulmonary vein isolation remains the key to ablation in atrial fibrillation, important advancements in the development of balloon materials are needed. Balloon compliance should allow antral coverage plus electrical monitoring while bringing pulmonary vein flow to a complete stop.

Acknowledgments

I would like to express my gratitude to my colleague Dr. Johannes Heintze for his decade-long support of our joint efforts in treating patients with cryoablation techniques and in advancing the science of cryoablation for managing atrial fibrillation.

I thank Mrs. Cordula Kreft, Mrs. Birgit Wellmann, and Mrs. Simone Rolfsmeier for maintaining the databases and for their involvement in follow-ups.

For making arrangements to have this manuscript, the illustrations, and the figure legends translated, I express many thanks to Mrs. Astrid Kleemeyer, our research secretary.

 Interactive Case Studies related to this chapter can be found at this book's companion website, at **www.chancryoablation.com**

References

1. Haissaguerre M, Shah D, Jais P, *et al.* Electrophysiological breakthroughs from the left atrium to the pulmonary veins. Circulation. 2000;101:1409–17.
2. Cappato R, Negroni S, Pecora D, *et al.* Prospective assessment of late conduction recurrence across radiofrequency lesions producing electrical disconnection

at the pulmonary vein ostium in patients with atrial fibrillation. Circulation. 2003;108:1599–604.

3. Khairy P, Chauvet P, Lehmann J, et al. Lower incidence of thrombus formation with cryoenergy versus radiofrequency catheter ablation. Circulation 2003;107: 2045–50.

4. Baust JG, Gage AA. The molecular basis of cryosurgery. BJU Int. 2005;95:1187–91.

5. Sarabanda AV, Bunch TJ, Johnson SB, et al. Efficacy and safety of circumferential pulmonary vein isolation using a novel cryothermal balloon ablation system. J Am Coll Cardiol. 2005;46:1902–12.

6. Siklódy CH, Minners J, Allgeier M, et al. Pressure-guided cryoballoon isolation of the pulmonary veins for the treatment of paroxysmal atrial fibrillation. J Cardiovasc Electrophysiol. 2010;21:120–5.

7. Siklódy CH, Minners J, Allgeier M, et al. Cryoballoon pulmonary vein isolation guided by transesophageal echocardiography: novel aspects on an emerging ablation technique. J Cardiovasc Electrophysiol. 2009; 20:1197–202.

8. Nölker G, Heintze J, Gutleben KJ, et al. Cryoballoon pulmonary vein isolation supported by intracardiac echocardiography: integration of a non fluoroscopic imaging technique in atrial fibrillation ablation. J Cardiovasc Electrophysiol. 2010;21;1325–30.

9. Sorgente A, Chierchia GB, de Asmundis C, et al. Pulmonary vein ostium shape and orientation as possible predictors of occlusion in patients with drug-refractory paroxysmal atrial fibrillation undergoing cryoballoon ablation. Europace. 2011;13:205–12.

10. Vogt J, Heintze J, Gutleben KJ, et al. Impact of balloon size strategy on long term success in antral cryo isolation of pulmonary veins. Heart Rhythm. 2011;8; S195.

11. Chun KR, Schmidt B, Metzner A, et al. The "single big cryoballoon" technique for acute pulmonary vein isolation in patients with paroxysmal atrial fibrillation: a prospective observational single centre study. Eur Heart J. 2009;30:699–709.

12. Kuck KH, Fürnkranz A. Cryoballoon ablation of atrial fibrillation. J Cardiovasc Electrophysiol. 2010;21: 1427–31.

13. Chun KR, Fürnkranz A, Metzner A, et al. Cryoballoon pulmonary vein isolation with real-time recordings from the pulmonary veins. J Cardiovasc Electrophysiol. 2009;20:1203–10.

14. Dorwarth U, Schmidt M, Wankerl M, et al. Pulmonary vein electrophysiology during cryoballoon ablation as a predictor for procedural success. J Interv Card Electrophysiol. 2011;32:205–11.

15. Ahmed H, Neuzil P, Skoda J, et al. The permanency of pulmonary vein isolation using a balloon cryoablation catheter. J Cardiovasc Electrophysiol. 2010;21: 731–7.

16. Neumann T, Vogt J, Schumacher B, et al. Circumferential pulmonary vein isolation with the cryoballoon technique: results from a prospective 3-center study. J Am Coll Cardiol. 2008;52:273–8.

17. Malmborg H, Lönnerholm S, Blomström-Lundqvist C. Acute and clinical effects of cryoballoon pulmonary vein isolation in patients with symptomatic paroxysmal and persistent atrial fibrillation. Europace. 2008;10:1277–80.

18. Klein G, Oswald H, Gardiwal A, et al. Efficacy of pulmonary vein isolation by cryoballoon ablation in patients with paroxysmal atrial fibrillation. Heart Rhythm. 2008;5:802–6.

19. Van Belle Y, Janse P, Theuns D, et al. One year follow-up after cryoballoon isolation of the pulmonary veins in patients with paroxysmal atrial fibrillation. Europace. 2008;10:1271–6.

20. Franceschi F, Dubuc M, Guerra PG, et al. Diaphragmatic electromyography during cryoballoon ablation: a novel concept in the prevention of phrenic nerve palsy. Heart Rhythm. 2011;8:885–91.

21. Sauren LD, Van Belle Y, De Roy L, et al. Transcranial measurement of cerebral microembolic signals during endocardial pulmonary vein isolation: comparison of three different ablation techniques. J Cardiovasc Electrophysiol. 2009;20:1102–7.

22. Gaita F, Leclercq JF, Schumacher B, et al. Incidence of silent cerebral thromboembolic lesions after atrial fibrillation ablation may change according to technology used: comparison of irrigated radiofrequency, multipolar nonirrigated catheter and cryoballoon. J Cardiovasc Electrophysiol. 2011;22:961–8.

23. Neumann T, Kuniss M, Conradi G, et al. MEDAFI-Trial (Micro-Embolization during Ablation of Atrial Fibrillation): comparison of pulmonary vein isolation using cryoballoon technique vs. radiofrequency energy. Europace. 2011;13:37–44.

24. Herrera Siklódy C, Deneke T, Hocini M, et al. Incidence of asymptomatic intracranial embolic events after pulmonary vein isolation: comparison of different atrial fibrillation ablation technologies in a multicenter study. J Am Coll Cardiol. 2011;58:681–8.

25. Wetzel U, Heintze J, Dorszewski A, et al. Long term follow up MRI angiographies before and after pulmonary vein isolation using a cryoballoon. Eur Heart J. 2008;29(Suppl. 1):412.

26. Packer DL, Irwin JM, Champagne J, et al. Cryoballoon ablation of pulmonary veins for paroxysmal atrial fibrillation: first results of the North American Arctic Front STOP-AF pivotal trial. J Am Coll Cardiol. 2010;55:E3015–6.

27. Thomas D, Katus HA, Voss F. Asymptomatic pulmonary vein stenosis after cryoballoon catheter ablation of paroxysmal atrial fibrillation. J Electrocardiol. 2011;44:473–6.

28. Pison L, La Meir M, Maessen J, *et al.* Extracardiac ice formation during cryoballoon technique for atrial fibrillation. Heart Rhythm. 2010;7:1518.

29. Herweg B, Ali R, Khan N, *et al.* Esophageal contour changes during cryoablation of atrial fibrillation. Pacing Clin Electrophysiol. 2009;32:711–6.

30. Ahmed H, Neuzil P, d'Avila A, *et al.* The esophageal effects of cryoenergy during cryoablation for atrial fibrillation. Heart Rhythm. 2009;6:962–9.

31. Fürnkranz A, Chun KR, Metzner A, *et al.* Esophageal endoscopy results after pulmonary vein isolation using the single big cryoballoon technique. J Cardiovasc Electrophysiol. 2010;21:869–74.

32. Yokoyama K, Nakagawa H, Seres KA, *et al.* Canine model of esophageal injury and atrial-esophageal fistula after applications of forward-firing high-intensity focused ultrasound and side-firing unfocused ultrasound in the left atrium and inside the pulmonary vein. Circ Arrhythm Electrophysiol. 2009;2:41–9.

33. Stöckigt F, Schrickel JW, Andrié R, *et al.* Atrioesophageal fistula after cryoballoon pulmonary vein isolation. J Cardiovasc Electrophysiol. 2012;23:1254–7. doi:10.1111/j.1540-8167.2012.02324.x

34. van Opstal JM, Timmermans C, Blaauw Y, *et al.* Bronchial erosion and hemoptysis after pulmonary vein isolation by cryoballoon ablation. Heart Rhythm. 2011;8:1459.

35. Cappato R, Calkins H, Chen SA, *et al.* Updated worldwide survey on the methods, efficacy, and safety of catheter ablation for human atrial fibrillation. Circ Arrhythm Electrophysiol. 2010;3:32–8.

36. Kojodjojo P, O'Neill MD, Lim PB, *et al.* Pulmonary venous isolation by antral ablation with a large cryoballoon for treatment of paroxysmal and persistent atrial fibrillation: medium-term outcomes and non-randomised comparison with pulmonary venous isolation by radiofrequency ablation. Heart. 2010;96:1379–84.

37. Andrade JG, Khairy P, Guerra PG, *et al.* Efficacy and safety of cryoballoon ablation for atrial fibrillation: a systematic review of published studies. Heart Rhythm. 2011;8:1444–51.

38. Vogt J, Heintze J, Gutleben KJ, et al. Long-term outcomes after cryoballoon pulmonary vein isolation: results from a prospective study in 605 patients. J Am Coll Cardiol 2013;61:707–712.

CHAPTER 6

Prevention of Phrenic Nerve Palsy during Cryoballoon Ablation for Atrial Fibrillation

Marcin Kowalski

Staten Island University Hospital, Staten Island, NY, USA

Introduction

Injury to the right phrenic nerve is the most common complication associated with pulmonary vein (PV) isolation when using cryoenergy. The injury may range from transient impairment of diaphragmatic function to permanent phrenic nerve palsy (PNP). On account of the anatomical course of the phrenic nerve, injury to the nerve occurs more frequently during ablation of the right superior pulmonary vein (RSPV) than during ablation of the right inferior pulmonary vein (RIPV).[1]

The incidence of phrenic nerve injury (PNI) during cryoballoon ablation has been reported to be between 2% and 11%,[1-5] and a meta-analysis of 23 articles reported PNI in 6.38% of the cases.[6] In the majority of the cases, phrenic nerve function recovered within one year. In the Sustained Treatment of Paroxysmal Atrial Fibrillation (STOP AF) trial, a randomized trial comparing cryoballoon ablation with antiarrhythmic medications, there were 29 cases of PNI, of which 4 persisted after one year.[5] In the US Continued Access Protocol (CAP-AF) registry, 4 out of 71 cases (5.6%) had PNI, with complete resolution in 3 patients.[7] In comparison to the cryoballoon technique, during PV isolation using radiofrequency energy, PNI is a rare complication (0.48%) and is frequently associated with ablation of the right PV orifice, the superior vena cava (SVC), and the roof of the left atrial appendage.[8-10]

Anatomy

The phrenic nerve originates from the third, fourth, and fifth cervical nerves and provides the only motor supply to the diaphragm as well as sensation to the central tendon, mediastinal pleura, and pericardium. The nerve descends almost vertically along the right brachiocephalic vein and continues along the right anterolateral surface of the SVC (Figure 6.1). The phrenic nerve is separated from the SVC by only the pericardium at the anterolateral junction between the SVC and the right atrium.[11] The close proximity of the nerve to the SVC wall in this location can facilitate capture of the nerve while pacing from the lateral wall of the SVC. Descending the anterolateral wall of the SVC, the nerve veers posteriorly as it approaches the superior cavoatrial junction and follows in close proximity to the pulmonary veins before reaching

The Practice of Catheter Cryoablation for Cardiac Arrhythmias, First Edition. Edited by Ngai-Yin Chan.
© 2014 John Wiley & Sons, Ltd. Published 2014 by John Wiley & Sons, Ltd.

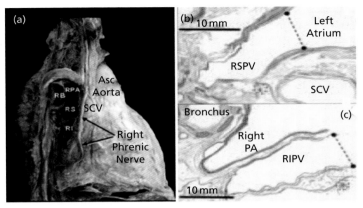

Figure 6.1. (a) Specimen shows the course of the phrenic nerve and the close anatomic relationship to other structures. RB: right bronchus; RI: right inferior; RM: right middle; RPA: right pulmonary artery; RS: right superior pulmonary veins; SCV: superior vena cava. (Source: Ho SY, Cabrera JA, Sanchez-Quintana D, 2012[11]. Reproduced with permission from Wolters Kluwer Health). (b) Histological sections through the RSPV and (c) the inferior pulmonary vein respectively. The right phrenic nerve (surrounded by dots) is adherent to the fibrous pericardium (thin red-green line). The broken lines indicate the pulmonary venous orifices. Note the myocardial sleeve (red) on the outer side of the RSPV. ICV: inferior vena cava; PA: pulmonary artery; RIPV: right inferior pulmonary vein; RSPV: right superior pulmonary vein; SCV: superior caval vein. (Masson's trichrome stain.) (Source: Sanchez-Quintana D, Cabrera JA, Climent V, Farre J, Weiglein A, Ho SY, 2005[12]. Reproduced with permission from John Wiley and Sons Ltd).

the diaphragm. Histologic examination of the transverse sections revealed that the phrenic nerve is, on average, located closer to the RSPV (2.1 ± 0.4 mm) than to the RIPV (3.2 ± 0.9 mm) (Figure 6.1).[12] The close proximity of the phrenic nerve to the RSPV renders it more vulnerable to injury during cryoballoon ablation of the RSPV then during ablation of the RIPV.

Mechanisms of phrenic nerve injury

The mechanisms of PNI during cryoballoon application are presumably multifactorial (Table 6.1). The mechanisms of cellular damage that are secondary to the cryoenergy application include ice crystal formation in the extracellular space, resulting in a hyperosmotic milieu in extravascular spaces that draws water from the cell, causing intracellular desiccation. As the temperature decreases, the extracellular crystals increase in number and cause mechanical damage to the cell membrane and organs. As the freezing continues, the intracellular crystals can form and cause further harm to the cell. A delayed direct cell injury may result from apoptosis, inflammation, coagulation necrosis of

Table 6.1. Mechanisms of phrenic nerve injury

Proximity of the phrenic nerve (PN) to the pulmonary vein (PV)
Distortion of the PV geometry by the balloon inflation
Excessive temperature
Duration of the freeze
Repetitive freeze-thaw cycle
Vasoconstriction, thrombosis, and ischemia caused by hypothermia
Previous injury to the nerve

the cell, and replacement fibrosis.[13,14] Vascular responses to cold temperature include vasoconstriction causing ischemia and circulatory stasis, which has also been shown to play an important role in cellular damage during cryotherapy.

The distance between the cryoballoon and the phrenic nerve plays an important role in the degree of damage to the nerve. The tissue is cooled with outward expansion in a concentric fashion from the cryoballoon surface touching the cardiac tissue.[15] The closer the phrenic nerve is to the atrial tissue adjoining the cryoballoon surface, the colder the temperatures are near the nerve, making nerve damage more likely. Okumura *et al.* showed in 10 dogs that balloon inflation at the PV orifice alters the geometry of the native RSPV endocardial surface and reduces the distance between the balloon and the phrenic nerve.[16] The inflated balloon surface extended outside the diameter of the original PV distortion is 5.6 ± 3.7 mm anteriorly and 2.7 ± 3.5 mm posteriorly. Furthermore, prominent distortions of the RSPV and the RSPV orifice moved the anatomic position of the phrenic nerve on average by 4.3 ± 2.9 mm in the anterior to lateral directions. The degree of anatomic distortion is amplified when the balloon is pushed slightly into the PV to minimize leaks.

The temperature achieved during a freeze and the duration of cryoapplication can make a significant difference in the incidence of PNI and the recovery of the nerve function. Colder temperatures achieved during the freeze expand the cold front further into the tissue, creating a deeper lesion and increasing the chance of reaching detrimental temperatures near the phrenic nerve. Assuming that the balloon has good contact with the tissue at $-30\,^{\circ}\text{C}$ and remains in contact for several minutes, the $0\,^{\circ}\text{C}$ isotherm will be located 3 mm deep. If the temperature, however, decreases to $-90\,^{\circ}\text{C}$, the isotherm will be roughly 1.4 cm deep.[17] Exposure to freezing temperatures can induce responses in the tissues that vary from inflammation during minor cold injury to tissue destruction during greater cold injury.[14] Based on previous research, peripheral nerves lose function when exposed to a temperature of 0 to $-5\,^{\circ}\text{C}$. The function returns when the temperature rises if the sheath is intact.[18,19] Fast freezing of tissue occurs only very close to the balloon. Most of the frozen volume of tissue experiences slow cooling, which is not as lethal to cells as fast cooling. Colder temperatures may be achieved when the cryoballoon is advanced deeper into the PV. Therefore, it is imperative to position the balloon as antral as possible. As the duration of the cryoablation is extended, the size of the lesion continues to expand and the affected area becomes larger. Animals that were randomized to longer application duration demonstrated a higher degree of cell destruction and fibrotic content.[20] Lesion size continues to expand during the cryoablation application, which can last up to 2–3 minutes.[15] Beazley

and colleagues showed that the length of the nerve regeneration period or the duration of the nerve palsy is predictable based on the distance between the site of the cryolesion and the nerve and the duration in which the nerve is exposed to cryoenergy.[21] Therefore, if the application of cryoenergy is stopped early enough to prevent prolonged exposure of the phrenic nerve to lethal temperatures, the injury to the nerve can be reversed.

Other mechanisms of PNI include vasoconstriction and decreased blood flow induced by hypothermia. The decrease in blood supply to the nerve can intensify the injury.[22–25] Also, a repetitive freeze-thaw cycle can be more destructive to the tissue, as the conduction of the cold front through the tissue is faster with repeated freezing and larger crystals may result from the fusion of previously formed crystals.[22,26] When tissue cooling is faster and the volume of cellular necrosis increases, the PV can be injured more rapidly.[14] Furthermore, a phrenic nerve with previously compromised functioning (either mechanically from previous ablations or surgery or from neurological diseases such as myasthenia gravis or Guillain–Barré syndrome) is at an increased risk for further injury by any of the mechanisms described here.[27] In these cases, special attention needs to be given and precautions need to be taken during the ablation to prevent further injury to the nerve.

Pacing the phrenic nerve

Currently, there is no reliable method that can predict PNI prior to the procedure. To prevent permanent PNP, it is essential to continuously monitor phrenic nerve function during the cryoenergy application in both the right superior and right inferior pulmonary veins. The phrenic nerve function is monitored by advancing a pacing catheter into the SVC, capturing the phrenic nerve above the level of the cryoballoon, and monitoring the intensity of the diaphragmatic excursions (Figure 6.2). The best site at which to capture the phrenic nerve is in the anterior-lateral portion of the SVC near the atrial–SVC junction because at that location, the phrenic nerve is separated from the SVC wall by only the pericardium.

It is imperative that short-acting paralytics are administered only during the induction of general

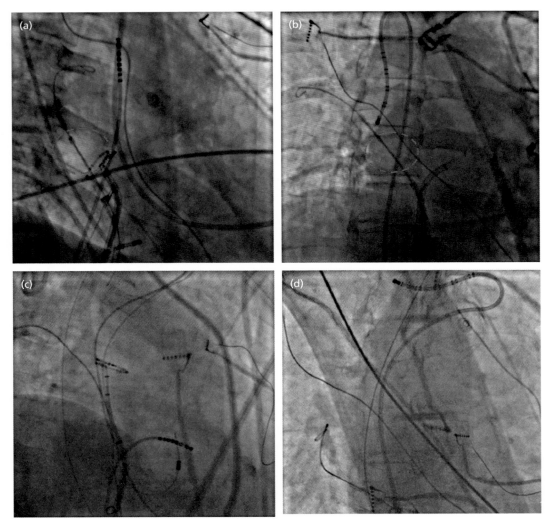

Figure 6.2. Position of different catheters in the superior vena cava (SVC) to facilitate capture of the phrenic nerve. (a) Deflectable octapolar catheter (Biosense Webster Inc., CA, United States) located on the lateral wall of the SVC. Notice that the phrenic nerve is captured above the cryoballoon. (b) Deflectable decapolar catheter (Biosense Webster Inc.) prolapsed into the SVC. Notice the retroflexed curve for better stability. (c) Lasso Circular Mapping Catheter (Biosense Webster Inc.) and a more distal portion of the decapolar catheter advanced distal in the SVC (d) for stable phrenic nerve capture.

anesthesia in order to allow adequate time for the paralytic effect to abate prior to ablation of the right-sided PV. A paralytic effect can hinder accurate monitoring of the phrenic nerve function, delay cryoablation of the right-sided vein, and mask PNP during the ablation. If the paralytic effect lingers, neostigmine may be used as a reversal agent.

Different catheters might be used to pace the phrenic nerve (Figure 6.2). However, the stability of the catheter and the reliable capture of the phrenic nerve are essential during pacing. A sudden loss of capture due to catheter movement may mimic PNI. Conversely, the operator may be misled by loss of capture if he or she assumes the catheter was displaced, but in reality PNI had occurred. The failure to recognize PNI can delay termination of the ablation and cause permanent phrenic nerve damage. A deflectable His catheter or coronary sinus catheter can provide satisfactory stability and pacing. Prolapsing the coronary sinus catheter into the SVC and retroflexing the tip can help stabilize the catheter and facilitate pacing (Figure 6.2). A circular mapping catheter (Lasso, Biosense Webster Inc., CA, USA) advanced into the SVC may provide excellent stability and capture; however, it requires a long sheath and adds extra cost. The closer the phrenic nerve is captured near the cryoballoon, the higher the chance of PNI. However, capturing the phrenic nerve at a further distance from the balloon does not eliminate the chance of PNI. Prior to ablation, it is helpful to obtain a phrenic nerve pacing threshold. The stimulation of the phrenic nerve should be carried out at twice the pacing threshold. A high current strength can potentially

overcome early nerve injury and conceal damage to the nerve.[28] The phrenic nerve should be paced at an interval between 40 and 60 bpm. A slower pacing rate can delay the detection of PNP, and a rapid pacing rate can prematurely fatigue the diaphragm.[29]

Monitoring of the phrenic nerve function

Fluoroscopy and palpation

During the cryoenergy application, multiple modalities are currently utilized to monitor phrenic nerve function while pacing the nerve from the SVC (Table 6.2). Continued or intermittent fluoroscopy of the right diaphragm during phrenic nerve pacing can accurately diagnose the decrease in phrenic nerve

Table 6.2. Comparison of different strategies for monitoring phrenic nerve palsy during cryoballoon ablation

Method	Description	Advantages	Disadvantages
Fluoroscopy	Direct visualization of diaphragmatic motion with fluoroscopy	• A sensitive method for monitoring diaphragmatic motion • Used to evaluate reliable phrenic nerve capture prior to cryoablation	• Additional radiation exposure to the patient and the operator • Does not predict phrenic nerve injury (PNI)
Palpation	Palpation of diaphragmatic excursion	• Reliable and simple to apply method for monitoring diaphragmatic motion	• Requires extra staff member • The strength of diaphragmatic excursion may change with respiration
Electromyography	Recording of diaphragmatic compound motor action potential (CMAP) by two standard surface electrodes positioned across the diaphragm	• Earliest detection of phrenic nerve injury • The method is simple and easily applicable. • The only technique that may predict PNI	• CMAP signals might be susceptible to respiratory variations. • The baseline amplitude must be adequate. • Affected by paralytic agents
Auditory cardiotocograph	Decrescendo pitch on fetal heart monitor (placed across patient's chest to detect diaphragmatic contractions)	• An auditory cue to the operator • May alert operator of PNI prior to palsy	• Extra equipment placed in the lab • May be difficult to record in obese patients
Intracardiac echocardiogram (ICE)	Direct visualization of strength of diaphragmatic excursion	• Less radiation exposure to the patient and the operator	• Requires additional venous access and the intracardiac ultrasound
Capnography	Direct monitoring of the CO_2 concentration in the respiratory gases and plotting a waveform of the expiratory CO_2 against time	• Used as an adjunctive technique to monitor phrenic nerve function	• Provides only indirect evidence of phrenic nerve function

function by observing the diminished diaphragmatic excursion. Although this method provides direct visualization of the diaphragmatic motion, it also exposes the patient and operator to additional radiation and, because of this, is the least used approach. Another technique utilized to monitor phrenic nerve function is palpation of the diaphragmatic excursion during phrenic nerve pacing. During phrenic nerve pacing, diaphragmatic contractions are sensed by placing the hand over the right diaphragm and below the costal margin and palpating every excursion. Weakening of the diaphragmatic contraction can indicate PNI. This method is easily applicable, but the strength of the diaphragmatic contraction can vary with respiration, which can misleadingly indicate PNI.

Intracardiac echocardiography and fetal heart monitoring

Intracardiac echocardiography (ICE) may be utilized to continuously visualize the motion of the liver with its capsule and indirectly image the contraction of the diaphragm during phrenic nerve pacing.[30] The ICE transducer (AcuNav, Acuson Siemens Corp., CA, United States) is positioned at the level of the diaphragm and pointed at the liver (Figure 6.3). The decrease in intensity of liver movement from the diaphragmatic excursion can be

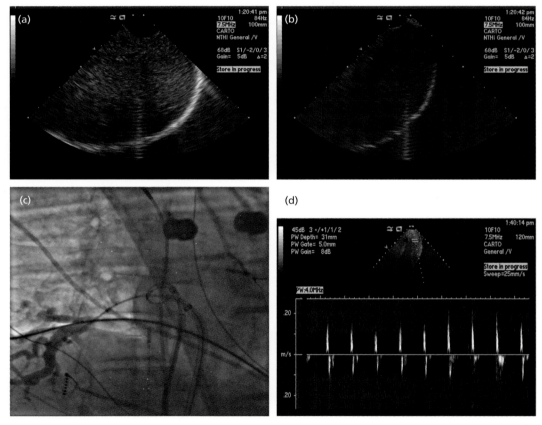

Figure 6.3. Intracardiac echocardiographic images of the diaphragm and the liver during phrenic nerve pacing showing the diaphragm (a) relaxing and (b) contracting. (c) Fluoroscopy image showing position of intracardiac echocardiography catheter (arrow) at the level of diaphragm. (Source: Lakhani M, Saiful F, Bekheit S, Kowalski M, 2012[30]. Reproduced with permission from John Wiley and Sons Ltd). (d) Pulse Doppler of the liver motion during phrenic nerve pacing. Notice the change in the amplitude of the velocity due to respiratory variation (private communication from Dr. Raman Mitra).

easily observed and can correlate with PNP (Figure 6.3).[30] If the entire liver cannot be easily visualized, a pulse wave Doppler can be placed on the liver to observe the liver exertions as a Doppler waveform. A decrease in Doppler amplitude can indicate PNP (Figure 6.3). ICE is an easily applicable tool for continuous direct diaphragmatic visualization without the use of fluoroscopy, thereby significantly minimizing radiation to both the patient and the operator.

Another method to monitor for PNI is to place an external Doppler fetal heart monitor at the right costal margin and listen for a change in pitch of the diaphragmatic contraction. A fetal heart monitor uses the Doppler effect to provide an audible simulation of diaphragmatic contractions. As the strength of the diaphragmatic contraction decreases during phrenic nerve pacing, an easily recognizable change in pitch can be perceived. The fetal heart monitor can provide an auditory cue to the physician and staff of possible PNI, detectable even in a busy lab (Audio Clip 6.1).

Diaphragmatic compound motor action potential

A method found to detect the earliest changes to phrenic nerve function induced by cryoballoon ablation is diaphragmatic electromyography (EMG). During phrenic nerve pacing, a reproducible supramaximal diaphragmatic compound motor action potential (CMAP) can be reliably recorded, providing valuable information about phrenic nerve function. The initial description of electrical activity of the diaphragm by surface electrodes over the lower intercostal spaces was made by Davis in 1967 in both healthy patients and those with peripheral neuropathy.[31] The location of the electrode yielding the largest diaphragm CMAP amplitude was 5 cm superior to the xiphoid and 16 cm from the xiphoid along the right costal margin.[32] The CMAP recordings of the phrenic nerve provided useful information on phrenic nerve function in patients with neuromuscular disorders that affect phrenic nerve conduction, especially in the intensive care unit for patients who are difficult to wean from the ventilator.[33,34]

The CMAP is a polyphasic signal composed of four intervals: onset latency, peak latency, dura-

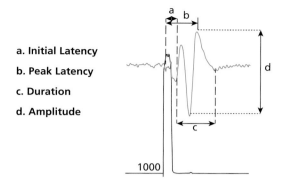

a. **Initial Latency**

b. **Peak Latency**

c. **Duration**

d. **Amplitude**

Figure 6.4. A polyphasic compound motor action potential (CMAP) recorded at a sweep speed of 200 mm/s speed was magnified to demonstrate the following intervals: (a) onset latency, (b) peak latency, (c) duration, and (d) amplitude. (Source: Franceschi F, Dubuc M, Guerra PG et al, 2011[35]. Reproduced with permission from Elsevier, Copyright © 2011 Elsevier).

tion, and amplitude (Figure 6.4).[31,35] Franceschi *et al.* examined the feasibility of recording diaphragmatic CMAPs during cryoballoon ablation and defined characteristic CMAP changes that herald phrenic nerve paralysis in the canine model.[35] In 16 canines, a 6-F steerable decapolar catheter (Livewire, St. Jude Medical, MN, United States) with electrodes spaced 5 mm apart was placed in the distal esophagus to record CMAPs. Cryoablation was performed with a 23 mm cryoballoon during phrenic nerve pacing at a site most likely to result in PNI. The study found that reduction of the CMAP amplitude was the earliest indication of PNI (Figure 6.5). At the time of earliest reduction in diaphragmatic excursion by fluoroscopy, the CMAP amplitude decreased by 48.1% ± 15.4%. In comparison, the maximum reduction in CMAP amplitude produced by cryoballoon applications not associated with a reduction in diaphragmatic excursion was 15.1% ± 12.1% ($P < 0.0001$). A 30% reduction in CMAP amplitude yielded the best discriminatory profile in predicting impaired diaphragmatic excursion with a sensitivity of 94.7% and a specificity of 87.5%. A 30% reduction in CMAP amplitude occurred at a mean of 33 ± 21 seconds. The average time interval from the 30% reduction in CMAP amplitude preceded the first fluoroscopic evidence of palsy by 6 sec and palpation by 31 sec. Another

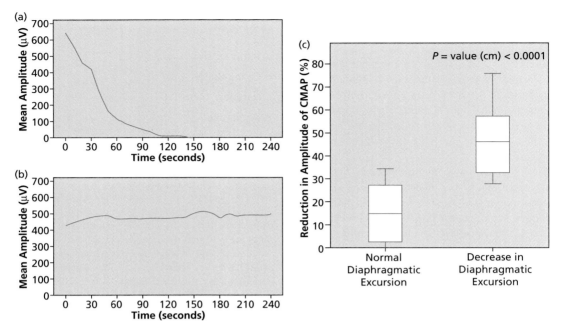

Figure 6.5. Amplitude of the phrenic compound motor action potential (CMAP) during a cryoballoon ablation that did (a) and did not (b) result in hemidiaphragmatic paralysis. In (a), an exponential reduction in the amplitude of the CMAP is noted during lesions that resulted in phrenic nerve paralysis, with the largest effect during the first minute. In contrast, (b) portrays relatively stable CMAP amplitudes during cryoballoon ablation applications that did not result in hemidiaphragmatic paralysis. (c) Boxplots of the reduction in CMAP amplitude that is associated with lesions that did not result in a reduction in diaphragmatic excursion (left) compared with lesions that paralyzed the right phrenic nerve at the time of first perceptible reduction in diaphragmatic motion (right). Lower and upper edges of the box indicate lower and upper quartiles. The line in the box represents the median value. Lower and upper bars indicate the 10th and 90th percentiles. (Source: Franceschi F, Dubuc M, Guerra PG et al, 2011[35]. Reproduced with permission from Elsevier, Copyright © 2011 Elsevier).

study randomized 32 canines to conventionally monitor either phrenic nerve function during cryoballoon ablation of the RSPV or monitoring the nerve with diaphragmatic CMAP and ceasing ablation upon a 30% decrease in CMAP amplitude.[36] The early termination of cryoablation guided by decrease in CMAP amplitude resulted in a lower rate of acute clinical PNI and a trend toward greater potential for recovery in the event of PNP. The injury to the phrenic nerve might be axonal in nature,[36] which is consistent with previous work in peripheral axonal neuropathy showing that a loss in CMAP amplitude reflects a disruption in axonal integrity. On the other hand, the slowing of conduction velocity or prolongation of latency implies demyelination.[28] Also, focal distal cooling has a

more pronounced effect on amplitude, and diffuse cooling has a more profound effect on conduction velocity.[28]

Franceschi et al. described the first clinical application of diaphragmatic CMAPs recorded with surface electrodes to prevent cryoballoon ablation–induced PNP.[37] Cryoablation was interrupted with forcible balloon deflation upon a 20% reduction in CMAP amplitude, which is when diaphragmatic excursion remained intact. A transient reduction in hemidiaphragmatic motion ensued, which fully recovered within a minute.

Lakhani et al. evaluated diaphragmatic CMAPs that were recorded on modified lead I (Figure 6.6) in 44 consecutive patients who underwent cryoballoon ablation.[38] Lead I was modified by placing

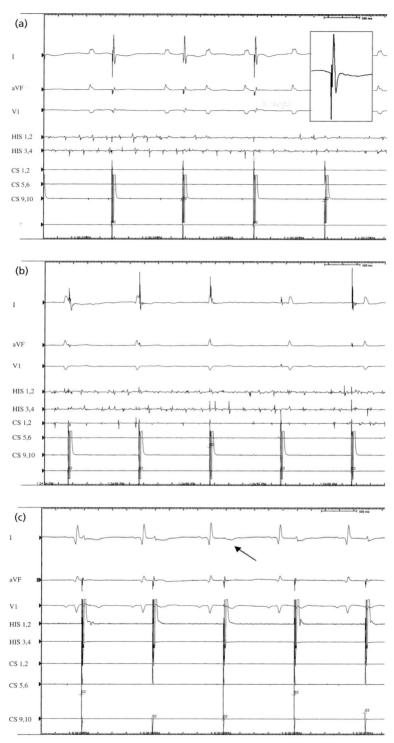

Figure 6.6. (a) Recordings of the diaphragmatic compound motor action potential (CMAP) during pacing from the coronary sinus (CS) catheter at 60 bpm located in the superior vena cava (SVC). The magnified CMAP recordings are located in the upper left corner. Notice the normal sinus rhythm in the background dissociated from the pacing. (b) An example of noncapturing of the phrenic nerve during pacing from SVC. (c) An example of intermittent phrenic nerve capture during pacing from SVC. Unintentionally, the patient received a paralytic agent 10 min prior to pacing. Notice the low amplitude of CMAP and one noncaptured beat (arrow). His: His bundle.

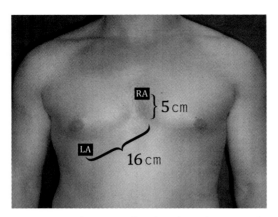

Figure 6.7. Configuration of surface electrodes to record diaphragmatic compound motor action potential on modified lead I. The right arm (RA) surface electrode is placed 5 cm above the xiphoid, and the left arm (LA) surface electrode is placed 16 cm from the xiphoid down the costal margin.

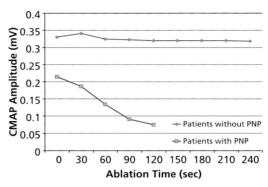

Figure 6.8. A graph of CMAP amplitude recorded using modified lead I during cryoballoon ablation in patients with and without phrenic nerve palsy (PNP). With sharp reduction in the amplitude on the beginning of the ablation. The results are comparable with the data presented by [35]. (Source: Lakhani M, Saiful F, Goyal N, Bekheit S, Kowalski M, 2012[38]. Reproduced with permission from Elsevier, Copyright © 2012 Elsevier).

the standard surface right-arm electrocardiogram (ECG) electrode 5 cm above the xiphoid and the left-arm ECG electrode 16 cm along the right costal margin (Figure 6.7). In the study, three (6.8%) patients developed PNI during a total of 170 cryo-balloon applications to 86 right-sided PVs. The minimal average CMAP amplitude during the freeze (0.31 ± 0.19 mV) did not significantly change in patients without PNP from the initial average CMAP amplitude (0.33 ± 0.2 mV) ($P = 0.58$). However, in patients with PNP, there was a sharp drop in the average CMAP amplitude from 0.22 ± 0.01 mV to 0.07 ± 0.01 mV ($P < 0.001$) (Figure 6.8). A decrease of CMAP amplitude during the cryoenergy application greater than 35% of the initial amplitude predicted PNI, a threshold that is consistent with prior results.[38] The initial CMAP amplitude prior to ablation was lower in patients with PNP than in patients without PNP. When comparing the initial CMAP amplitude before the first and the second applications of the cryoballoon in patients without PNP, the amplitude decreased in almost 50% of patients, and the decrease in amplitude was more evident in the RSPV. The decreased CMAP amplitude prior to the second freeze can indicate an initial injury to the nerve, which is consistent with the freeze-thaw hypothesis of cryoinjury.[17,26]

Monitoring the phrenic nerve function using diaphragmatic CMAP can effectively decrease PNI. The amplitude of CMAPs may be affected by respiration or body habitués. Adjusting the electrode more superiorly may help obtain a better signal in obese patients as the viscera pushes up on the diaphragm when the patient is lying supine.

Using capnography as an adjunctive tool for monitoring phrenic nerve function

A capnogram directly monitors the concentration of CO_2 in the respiratory gases and plots a waveform of the expiratory CO_2 against time. Phrenic nerve pacing causes an unnatural contraction of the diaphragm that translates into an interrupted pattern of CO_2 concentration (Figure 6.9). When the phrenic nerve is injured, the pattern changes to a conventional waveform associated with normal inhalation and exhalation; as the right diaphragm is not contracting, the left diaphragm continues to assist in normal gas exchange. This method should be used as an adjunctive technique to monitor phrenic nerve function and not as a primary method as it provides only indirect evidence of phrenic nerve function.

Recommendations

PNI is a complication associated with cryoballoon ablation that can be avoided with appropriate planning and monitoring (Table 6.3). It is vital to discuss the importance of phrenic nerve monitoring with the laboratory staff and anesthesiologist prior to the beginning of the case. During the ablation of the right-sided PVs, the laboratory staff should be attentive to any signs of phrenic nerve dysfunction and trained to stop ablation immediately. If the patient is intubated, the anesthesiologist must

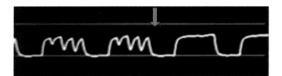

Figure 6.9. On the left of the figure, a capnogram waveform is shown during right phrenic nerve pacing. Each notch during the plateau represents contraction of the diaphragm. The arrow indicates development of phrenic nerve palsy and the immediate change in waveform to a normal breathing pattern.

know not to use any long-acting paralytic agents during the case or administer extra doses of the paralytic agents preceding ablation of the right-sided PV. A short-acting paralytic agent can be administered at the beginning of the case to facilitate intubation as the effect of the agent will dissipate during the case before pacing of the phrenic nerve is required.

Inflation of the balloon at the PV orifice distorts the geometry of the native PV endocardial surface and reduces the distance between the balloon surface and the phrenic nerve, despite the absence of the balloon's migration into the vein.[16] The degree of anatomic distortion can also be amplified when the balloon is pushed slightly into the PV to maximize the occlusion. Reducing the distance between the balloon and the phrenic nerve increases the chance of injury to the nerve. Therefore, it is imperative to inflate the balloon outside the PV and maintain the balloon as antral as possible during the ablation to prevent anatomic distortion of the PV orifice. PNI may be more common with the use of the 23 mm balloon, which results in more distal PV cryoablation. In early experiences with cryoballoons,

Table 6.3. Recommendations to prevent phrenic nerve injury

- Discuss the importance of phrenic nerve monitoring with the laboratory staff and anesthesiologist prior to the beginning of the case.
- If patient had prior CABG or valve replacement, perform inhalation and exhalation chest x-ray to exclude left diaphragm palsy. If left diaphragm palsy is present consider not to use cryoballoon to isolate the right PV as it may cause bilateral phrenic nerve palsy.
- Avoid long-acting paralytic agents during cryoballoon ablation if patient is intubated as it will prevent pacing of phrenic nerve and monitoring of its function.
- Inflate the balloon outside the pulmonary vein (PV) and maintain the balloon as antral as possible to prevent anatomic distortion of the PV orifice.
- Monitor the rate of temperature descent as a steep descent can indicate distal locating of the balloon.
- Vigorously monitor the phrenic nerve function by pacing the phrenic nerve from the superior vena cava (SVC) above the cryoballoon.
- Continuously pace the phrenic nerve from the SVC during ablation of both right superior pulmonary vein and right inferior pulmonary vein.
  - The stimulation of the PN should be carried out at twice the pacing threshold.
- Monitor phrenic nerve function by measuring it, feeling it, hearing it, or seeing it.
  - Measure the change in diaphragmatic compound motor action potential (CMAP) amplitude. A 30% reduction in CMAP amplitude yielded the most discriminatory cutoff value in predicting phrenic nerve injury.
  - Feel the excursion of the diaphragm by palpation.
  - Hear the change in tone of diaphragmatic excursion using a fetal heart monitor.
  - Visualize the motion of the liver and diaphragm by intracardiac echocardiography.
- Simultaneously employ the diaphragmatic CMAP amplitude and one or two other techniques to monitor phrenic nerve function.
- Immediately stop ablation at any signs of phrenic nerve injury.
  - Immediate deflation of the balloon may be initiated by pressing the emergency deflation button on the console.

Nuemann *et al.* reported 26 phrenic nerve palsies out of 346 patients (7.5%), 24 of which occurred when using the 23 mm balloon.[1] Injury to the right phrenic nerve can be minimized by using only the 28 mm cryoballoon;[3] the intentionally oversized balloon covers the proximal left atrial antrum region with as much distance from the phrenic nerve as possible.[12] Different signs or maneuvers may be utilized to successfully identify the suitable antral location of the balloon. When the balloon is appropriately engaged at the PV ostium (os), it takes the shape of an onion. However, when the balloon is deep inside the vein, both sides of the balloon become compressed, making the balloon more tubular to resemble a marshmallow (Figure 6.10). Some pulmonary veins, especially the RSPV, are funnel shaped, making the PV orifice potentially difficult to identify. To ensure that the balloon is not deep inside the vein, during contrast injection, the balloon can be slowly withdrawn to the left atrium until the contrast dissipates from the vein outlining the PV os (see Video Clip 6.1). This maneuver can outline the orifice of the vein that has difficult geometry and prevent balloon engagement deep inside the vein. Once the PV os is identified, the balloon can be slightly advanced forward and ablation can be initiated. When the cryoballoon is inflated and engaged at the PV os, an intracardiac echocardiogram can effectively identify the portion of the balloon located outside the PV. To prevent ablation inside the PV, at least 50% of the balloon's circumference should be visible outside the PV.

The rate of temperature descent and unusually low maximal temperature (usually below −60 °C) can prognosticate if the cryoballoon is located distal inside the PV. If the slope of temperature descent is very steep and the maximal temperature is reached quickly into the freeze, it is prudent to stop ablation and confirm if the balloon is not distal inside the PV.

See it, hear it, feel it, and measure it

Early detection of PNI and immediate termination of ablation are essential in the prevention of PNP. It is important to continuously monitor the phrenic nerve function by pacing the phrenic nerve above the cryoballoon during the ablation of both right-sided PVs. There is no reliable method to predict PNI; however, implementing vigorous monitoring of the nerve function can assure early detection and prevent permanent PNI. Since decrease in the CMAP amplitude is the earliest sign of detectable injury to the nerve (and is simple and easily applicable), it should be used as the major technique for

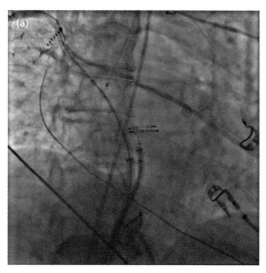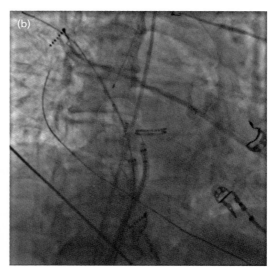

Figure 6.10. (a) A distal and (b) proximal location of the cryoballoon inside the right superior pulmonary veins in the same patient. Note that the balloon advanced distally inside the pulmonary vein takes a tubular shape, while a balloon positioned more antrally remains spherical.

monitoring in conjunction with one or two other methods. These methods include either palpation of the diaphragmatic excursion or movement of liver visualized on ICE or a fetal heart monitor. The amplitude of CMAP may be monitored by adjusting the caliper on the recording system 30% below the initial CMAP amplitude, as this yielded the most discriminatory cutoff value in predicting hemidiaphragmatic paralysis.[35,36,38] Once the amplitude decreases below the caliper line, ablation should be immediately terminated. Monitoring of the diaphragmatic motion by fluoroscopy may be employed to confirm phrenic nerve capture; however, due to the potential radiation exposure, this is the least favored method of monitoring phrenic nerve function.

Early discontinuation of ablation and warming of the tissue are vital in the prevention of permanent phrenic nerve damage. Reversible effects of cryothermal ablation were examined previously and are a function of temperature and duration.[20,22,26,35,37] Shorten the time the cell is exposed to a hypothermic insult and the warmer the temperature, the more rapidly the cell will recover.[39,40] A delay may be expected between cessation of the cryoapplication and the rewarming of the phrenic nerve, since the balloon temperature must reach +20°C before the cryoballoon deflates. Prior to complete balloon deflation, persistent occlusion of the pulmonary vein may slow the rewarming process and delay temperature rise. Therefore, an immediate deflation of the balloon may be initiated by pressing an emergency deflation button on the console to reestablish PV blood flow.

What to do when phrenic nerve injury occurs

Once PNI is detected by the methods described in this chapter, it is imperative to stop ablation immediately. Since the degree of the tissue injury is dependent on the temperature and the amount of time tissue is exposed to freezing temperatures, an early termination of ablation may prevent further damage and expedite recovery of the nerve function. If the injury to the phrenic nerve is recognized early and the ablation is terminated, the majority of the phrenic nerves recover in 12 months.[1,2,4] Inhalation and exhalation chest X-rays can confirm PNI after the procedure (Figure 6.11). The chest X-rays can be repeated a few weeks later to follow the phrenic nerve function if the patient continues to have symptoms. Since the late phase of cryoinjury involves inflammation,[26] steroids can be administered after the injury is detected. However, evidence does not exist to support this treatment.

Once injury to the nerve ensues during cryoballoon ablation, cryoenergy cannot be utilized to ablate the remaining right-sided PV because the phrenic nerve can no longer be monitored. Generally, by the time the PNI occurs, the PV is isolated because the cryoenergy has penetrated the tissue of the PV and completed the lesion. If the vein is not isolated or there is a remaining right-sided PV after

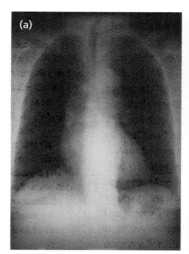 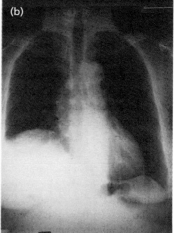

Figure 6.11. Inspiration chest X-rays performed (a) before and (b) after ablation. Patients suffered a right phrenic nerve palsy during the ablation as evident by an elevated right hemidiaphragm. (Source: Sacher F, Monahan KH, Thomas SP et al, 2006[9]. Reproduced with permission from Elsevier, Copyright © 2006 Elsevier).

PNP, the ablation ought to be completed using radiofrequency. Since PNI is more common during cryoballoon ablation of the RSPV, it might be feasible to ablate the RIPV before the RSPV.

Summary

PNI is the most common complication associated with circumferential ablation of the pulmonary veins using cryoballoon catheters to treat atrial fibrillation. The anatomic course of the phrenic nerve in close proximity to the right-sided pulmonary veins deems the nerve more susceptible to injury. The mechanism of the injury to the nerve is multifactorial and includes temperature, duration of the freezing, and anatomical distortion of the geometry of the native pulmonary vein's endocardial surface. There is no reliable method to predict PNI. However, the pacing of the phrenic nerve from the superior vena cava and vigorous monitoring of the nerve's integrity during cryoenergy application can detect the earliest sign of injury to the nerve. The decrease in diaphragmatic CMAP amplitude can precede diaphragmatic paralysis, and it should be used with one or two other methods to simultaneously monitor phrenic nerve function. The key to prevention of PNP is early recognition of injury to the nerve and immediate termination of ablation.

 Interactive Case Studies related to this chapter can be found at this book's companion website, at **www.chancryoablation.com**

References

1. Neumann T, Vogt J, Schumacher B, et al. Circumferential pulmonary vein isolation with the cryoballoon technique results from a prospective 3-center study. J Am Coll Cardiol. 2008;52:273–8.
2. Kojodjojo P, O'Neill MD, Lim PB, et al. Pulmonary venous isolation by antral ablation with a large cryoballoon for treatment of paroxysmal and persistent atrial fibrillation: medium-term outcomes and non-randomised comparison with pulmonary venous isolation by radiofrequency ablation. Heart. 2010;96: 1379–84.
3. Chun KR, Schmidt B, Metzner A, et al. The "single big cryoballoon" technique for acute pulmonary vein isolation in patients with paroxysmal atrial fibrillation: a prospective observational single centre study. Eur Heart J. 2009;30:699–709.
4. Van BY, Janse P, Rivero-Ayerza MJ, et al. Pulmonary vein isolation using an occluding cryoballoon for circumferential ablation: feasibility, complications, and short-term outcome. Eur Heart J. 2007;28:2231–7.
5. Packer DL, Iwin J. Cryoballoon ablation of pulmonary veins for paroxysmal atrial fibrillation: first results of the North American Arctic Front STOP-AF pivotal trial. J Am Coll Cardiol. 2010;55:E3015–6.
6. Andrade JG, Khairy P, Guerra PG, et al. Efficacy and safety of cryoballoon ablation for atrial fibrillation: a systematic review of published studies. Heart Rhythm. 2011;8:1444–51.
7. Packer DL, Kowal R, Wheelan K, et al. Impact of experience on efficacy and safety of cryoballoon ablation for atrial fibrillation: outcomes of the STOP-AF continued access protocol. Heart Rhythm. 2011;8:S379.
8. Bunch TJ, Bruce GK, Mahapatra S, et al. Mechanisms of phrenic nerve injury during radiofrequency ablation at the pulmonary vein orifice. J Cardiovasc Electrophysiol. 2005;16:1318–25.
9. Sacher F, Monahan KH, Thomas SP, et al. Phrenic nerve injury after atrial fibrillation catheter ablation: characterization and outcome in a multicenter study. J Am Coll Cardiol. 2006;47:2498–503.
10. Bai R, Patel D, Di BL, et al. Phrenic nerve injury after catheter ablation: should we worry about this complication? J Cardiovasc Electrophysiol. 2006;17:944–8.
11. Ho SY, Cabrera JA, Sanchez-Quintana D. Left atrial anatomy revisited. Circ Arrhythm Electrophysiol. 2012;5:220–8.
12. Sanchez-Quintana D, Cabrera JA, Climent V, et al. How close are the phrenic nerves to cardiac structures? Implications for cardiac interventionalists. J Cardiovasc Electrophysiol. 2005;16:309–13.
13. Takamatsu H, Zawlodzka S. Contribution of extracellular ice formation and the solution effects to the freezing injury of PC-3 cells suspended in NaCl solutions. Cryobiology. 2006;53:1–11.
14. Gage AA, Baust J. Mechanisms of tissue injury in cryosurgery. Cryobiology. 1998;37:171–86.
15. Dubuc M, Roy D, Thibault B, et al. Transvenous catheter ice mapping and cryoablation of the atrioventricular node in dogs. Pacing Clin Electrophysiol. 1999;22:1488–98.
16. Okumura Y, Henz BD, Bunch TJ, et al. Distortion of right superior pulmonary vein anatomy by balloon catheters as a contributor to phrenic nerve injury. J Cardiovasc Electrophysiol. 2009;20:1151–7.
17. The principles of cryobiology. In: Khairy P, Dubuc M, editors. Cryoablation for cardiac arrhythmias. Montreal: Montreal Heart Institute; 2008. p. 13–21.

18. Whittaker DK. Mechanisms of tissue destruction following cryosurgery. Ann R Coll Surg Engl. 1984;66:313–8.
19. Gaster RN, Davidson TM, Rand RW, et al. Comparison of nerve regeneration rates following controlled freezing or crushing. Arch Surg. 1971;103:378–83.
20. Atienza F, Almendral J, Sanchez-Quintana D, et al. Cryoablation time-dependent dose-response effect at minimal temperatures (−80 degrees C): an experimental study. Europace. 2009;11:1538–45.
21. Beazley RM, Bagley DH, Ketcham AS. The effect of cryosurgery on peripheral nerves. J Surg Res. 1974;16:231–4.
22. Khairy P, Dubuc M. Transcatheter cryoablation part I: preclinical experience. Pacing Clin Electrophysiol. 2008;31:112–20.
23. Rabb JM, Renaud ML, Brandt PA, et al. Effect of freezing and thawing on the microcirculation and capillary endothelium of the hamster cheek pouch. Cryobiology. 1974;11:508–18.
24. Rothenborg HW. Cutaneous circulation in rabbits and humans before, during, and after cryosurgical procedures measured by xenon-133 clearance. Cryobiology. 1970;6:507–11.
25. Zacarian SA, Stone D, Clater M. Effects of cryogenic temperatures on microcirculation in the golden hamster cheek pouch. Cryobiology. 1970;7:27–39.
26. Gill W, Fraser J, Carter DC. Repeated freeze-thaw cycles in cryosurgery. Nature. 1968;219:410–3.
27. Basiri K, Dashti M, Haeri E. Phrenic nerve CMAP amplitude, duration, and latency could predict respiratory failure in Guillain-Barre syndrome. Neurosciences (Riyadh). 2012;17:57–60.
28. Gooch CL, Weimer LH. The electrodiagnosis of neuropathy: basic principles and common pitfalls. Neurol Clin. 2007;25:1–28.
29. Glenn WW, Phelps ML. Diaphragm pacing by electrical stimulation of the phrenic nerve. Neurosurgery. 1985;17:974–84.
30. Lakhani M, Saiful F, Bekheit S. et al. Use of intracardiac echocardiography for early detection of phrenic nerve injury during cryoballoon pulmonary vein isolation. J Cardiovasc Electrophysiol. 2012;23:874–6.
31. Davis JN. Phrenic nerve conduction in man. J Neurol Neurosurg Psychiatry. 1967;30:420–6.
32. Dionne A, Parkes A, Engler B, et al. Determination of the best electrode position for recording of the diaphragm compound muscle action potential. Muscle Nerve. 2009;40:37–41.
33. Bolton CF. Neuromuscular abnormalities in critically ill patients. Intensive Care Med. 1993;19:309–10.
34. Zifko UA, Zipko HT, Bolton CF. Clinical and electrophysiological findings in critical illness polyneuropathy. J Neurol Sci. 1998;159:186–93.
35. Franceschi F, Dubuc M, Guerra PG, et al. Diaphragmatic electromyography during cryoballoon ablation: a novel concept in the prevention of phrenic nerve palsy. Heart Rhythm. 2011;8:885–91.
36. Andrade JG, Dubuc M, Guerra PG, et al. Comparison between standard monitoring and diaphragmatic electromyography for the prevention of phrenic nerve palsy during pulmonary vein isolation with a novel cryoballoon catheter. Heart Rhythm. 2012;9:S321–42.
37. Franceschi F, Dubuc M, Guerra PG, et al. Phrenic nerve monitoring with diaphragmatic electromyography during cryoballoon ablation for atrial fibrillation: the first human application. Heart Rhythm. 2011;8:1068–71.
38. Lakhani M, Saiful F, Goyal N, et al. Recording of diaphragmatic electromyograms during cryoballoon ablation for atrial fibrillation can accurately predict phrenic nerve palsy. Heart Rhythm. 2012;9:S387.
39. Lister JW, Hoffman BF, Kavaler F. Reversible cold block of the specialized cardiac tissues of the unanaesthetized dog. Science. 1964;145:723–5.
40. Lemola K, Dubuc M, Khairy P. Transcatheter cryoablation part II: clinical utility. Pacing Clin Electrophysiol. 2008;31:235–44.

CHAPTER 7

Linear Isthmus Ablation for Atrial Flutter: Catheter Cryoablation versus Radiofrequency Catheter Ablation

Gregory K. Feld and Navinder Sawhney

University of California, San Diego, CA and Sulpizio Family Cardiovascular Center, La Jolla, CA, USA

Introduction

Typical (and reverse typical) atrial flutter (AFL) may cause severe symptoms or serious complications, including stroke, myocardial infarction, and occasionally a tachycardia-induced cardiomyopathy. In addition, AFL is often medically refractory. Since the electrophysiologic substrate underlying AFL is now well established, and in view of its relative pharmacological resistance, catheter ablation has emerged as a safe and effective first-line treatment. While radiofrequency catheter ablation (RFCA) of AFL has a relatively high long-term success rate (>95%), it can cause complications, including cardiac perforation and tamponade, and it is associated with significant pain during ablation. Catheter cryoablation may therefore have some inherent advantages over RFCA for ablation of AFL. This chapter will review the role of RFCA versus catheter cryoablation for treatment of typical (and reverse typical) AFL.

Atrial flutter terminology

Due to the varied terminology used to describe human AFL in the past, the Working Group of Arrhythmias of the European Society of Cardiology and the North American Society of Pacing and Electrophysiology (now the Heart Rhythm Society) published a consensus document in 2001 to standardize terminology for AFL.[1] The terminology recommended by this working group to describe cavo-tricuspid isthmus (CTI)-dependent AFL, with either a counterclockwise or clockwise direction around the tricuspid valve annulus, is typical and reverse typical AFL, respectively.[1]

Pathophysiologic mechanisms of AFL

Typical and reverse typical AFL (Figure 7.1a and 7.1b) have been shown to be due to macro-reentry, in either a counterclockwise (typical) or clockwise (reverse typical) direction around the tricuspid valve annulus.[2-7] Slow conduction has been shown to be present in the CTI, accounting for one-third to one-half of the AFL cycle length.[8-10] The CTI is anatomically bounded by the inferior vena cava and Eustachian ridge posteriorly and the tricuspid valve annulus anteriorly, which form lines of conduction block or barriers delineating a protected zone in the reentry circuit.[5,11-13] The path of the reentrant circuit outside the confines of the CTI consists of a

The Practice of Catheter Cryoablation for Cardiac Arrhythmias, First Edition. Edited by Ngai-Yin Chan.
© 2014 John Wiley & Sons, Ltd. Published 2014 by John Wiley & Sons, Ltd.

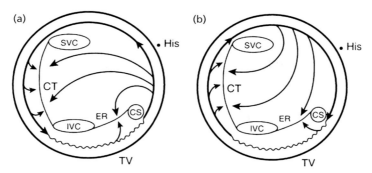

Figure 7.1. Schematic diagrams demonstrating the activation patterns in the typical (a) and reverse typical (b) forms of human type 1 atrial flutter (AFL), as viewed from below the tricuspid valve annulus looking up into the right atrium. In the typical form of AFL, the reentrant wavefront rotates counterclockwise in the right atrium, whereas in the reverse typical form reentry is clockwise. Note that the Eustachian ridge (ER) and crista terminalis (CT) form lines of block, and that an area of slow conduction (wavy line) is present in the isthmus between the inferior vena cava (IVC) and Eustachian ridge and the tricuspid valve annulus. CS: coronary sinus ostium, His: His bundle, SVC: superior vena cava. (Source: Adapted from Feld GK, Srivatsa U, Hoppe B, 2006[52]. Reproduced with permission from Elsevier, Copyright © 2006, Elsevier).

broad activation wavefront in the interatrial septum and right atrial free wall around the crista terminalis and the tricuspid valve annulus.[11–14]

Slow conduction in the CTI may be caused by anisotropic fiber orientation,[2] [8–10,15,16] which may also predispose to the development of unidirectional block in the CTI and account for the observation that typical AFL is more likely to be induced when pacing from the coronary sinus ostium, and conversely reverse typical AFL is more likely to be induced when pacing from the low lateral right atrium.[17–19] The predominant clinical presentation is typical AFL, likely because the triggers commonly arise from the left atrium in the form of premature atrial contractions or nonsustained atrial fibrillation,[20] which conduct into the CTI medially, resulting in clockwise unidirectional block and resultant initiation of typical AFL.

Electrocardiogram diagnosis of AFL

The surface 12-lead electrocardiogram (ECG) in typical AFL is usually diagnostic with an inverted saw-tooth F wave pattern in the inferior ECG leads II, III, and aVF; low-amplitude biphasic F waves in leads I and aVL; an upright F wave in precordial lead V1; and an inverted F wave in lead V6 (Figure

7.2a). In contrast, in reverse typical AFL the F wave pattern is less specific, with a sine wave pattern in the inferior ECG leads (Figure 7.2b). However, since typical and reverse typical AFL utilize the same reentry circuit, just in opposite directions, their rates are usually similar. The determinants of the F wave pattern on ECG are dependent on activation of the left atrium, with the inverted F waves in typical AFL resulting from activation of the left atrium initially via the coronary sinus, and the upright F waves in reverse typical AFL resulting from activation of the left atrium initially via Bachman's bundle.[21,22] Following extensive left atrial ablation for AF, the F wave pattern in typical AFL may be significantly different from the characteristic saw-tooth pattern, due to the reduction in left atrial voltage after ablation and the change in activation pattern.[23]

Mapping of AFL

Despite the utility of the 12-lead ECG in diagnosing AFL, an electrophysiologic study utilizing mapping and entrainment should be done to confirm the underlying mechanism, if catheter ablation is to be successful. This is particularly true for reverse typical AFL, which is more difficult to diagnose

(a)

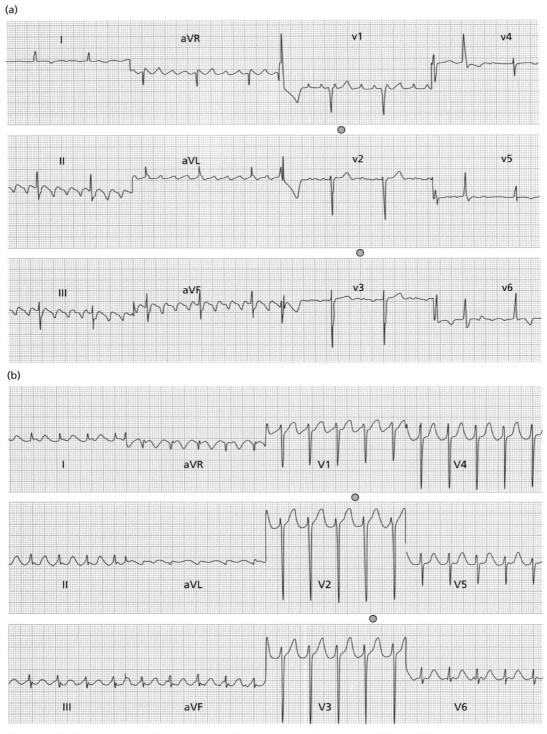

(b)

Figure 7.2. (a) 12-lead electrocardiogram recorded from a patient with typical atrial flutter (AFL). Note the typical saw-toothed pattern of inverted F waves in the inferior leads II, III, aVF. Typical AFL is also characterized by flat to biphasic F waves in I and aVL, respectively; an upright F wave in V1; and an inverted F wave in V6. (b) 12-lead electrocardiogram recorded from a patient with reverse typical AFL. The F wave in the reverse typical form of AFL has a less distinct sine wave pattern in the inferior leads. In this case, the F waves are upright in the inferior leads II, III, and aVF; biphasic in leads I, aVL, and V1; and upright in V6. (Source: Adapted from Feld GK, Srivvatsa U, Hoppe B, 2006[52]. Reproduced with permission from Elsevier, Copyright © 2006 Elsevier).

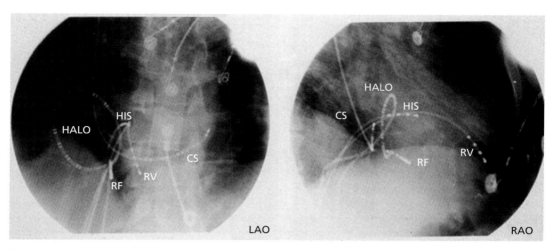

Figure 7.3. Left anterior oblique (LAO) and right anterior oblique (RAO) fluoroscopic projections showing the intracardiac positions of the right ventricular (RV), His bundle (HIS), coronary sinus (CS), Halo (HALO), and mapping and ablation catheter (RF). Note that the Halo catheter is positioned around the tricuspid valve annulus with the proximal electrode pair at the 1:00 o'clock position and the distal electrode pair at the 7:00 o'clock position in the LAO view. The mapping and ablation catheter is positioned in the sub-Eustachian isthmus, midway between the interatrial septum and low lateral right atrium, with the distal 8 mm ablation electrode near the tricuspid valve annulus. (Source: Adapted from Feld GK, Srivatsa U, Hoppe B, 2006[52]. Reproduced with permission from Elsevier, Copyright © 2006 Elsevier).

on ECG. For standard catheter mapping, multi-electrode catheters are positioned in the right atrium, His bundle region, and coronary sinus. To determine the endocardial activation sequence, a multipolar electrode-mapping catheter (e.g., Halo[TM] manufactured by Cordis-Webster, Inc., CA, United States) is commonly positioned in the right atrium around the tricuspid valve annulus (Figure 7.3). Recordings are then obtained from all electrodes during spontaneous or pacing-induced AFL and analyzed to determine right atrial activation sequence.[17,18] Typical and reverse typical AFL are characterized by a counterclockwise or clockwise activation pattern in the right atrium around the tricuspid valve annulus, respectively (Figure 7.4a and 7.4b), and demonstration of concealed entrainment during pacing from the CTI (Figure 7.5a and 7.5b) confirms the isthmus dependence of the reentry circuit.[5] Three-dimensional electroanatomical mapping may also be performed to diagnose and confirm the underlying mechanism of AFL, but it is not required for a successful outcome of ablation in most cases.

Radiofrequency catheter ablation of AFL

Catheter ablation of typical AFL has been performed most commonly with a steerable radiofrequency ablation catheter.[3,5-7,24-26] Although a variety of ablation catheters are currently available, we prefer to use a large-curve catheter, with a preshaped or steerable guiding sheath in order to ensure that the ablation electrode will reach the tricuspid valve annulus with good tissue contact. Catheters with either saline-cooled ablation electrodes or large distal ablation electrodes (i.e., 8–10 mm) are preferred. During ablation with saline-cooled catheters, a maximum power of 35–50 W and temperatures of 42–45 °C should be used initially, as powers above 50 W may lead to steam pops.[27-30] In contrast, large-tip (i.e., 8–10 mm) ablation catheters may require up to 100 W of power to achieve target temperatures of 50–70 °C, due to the greater energy-dispersive effects of the larger ablation electrode.[29,31-33]

The preferred target for ablation of typical AFL is the CTI.[3,5-7,24-30,32,33] The ablation catheter is

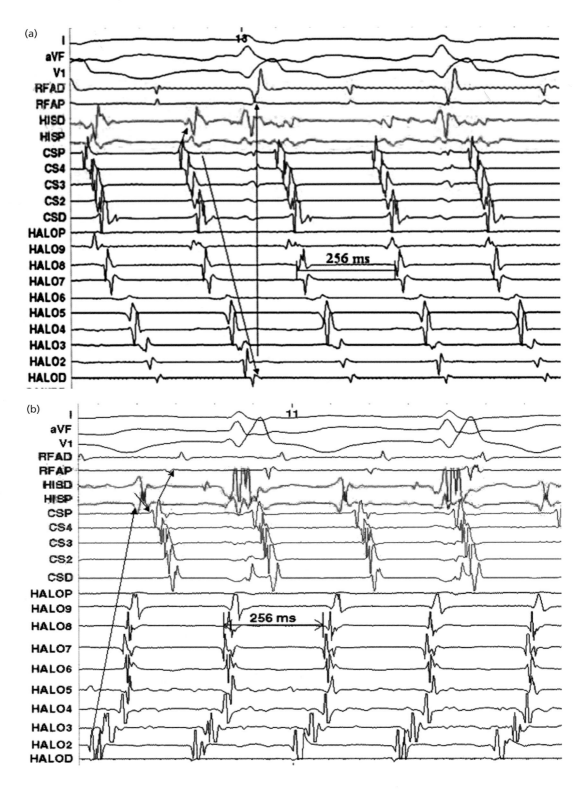

Figure 7.4. Endocardial electrograms from the mapping and ablation, Halo, CS, and His bundle catheters, and surface electrocardiogram (ECG) leads I and aVF, demonstrating (a) a counterclockwise (CCW) rotation of activation in the right atrium in a patient with typical atrial flutter (AFL), and (b) a clockwise (CW) rotation of activation in the right atrium in a patient with reverse typical AFL. The AFL cycle length was 256 msec for both CCW and CW forms. Arrows demonstrate the activation sequence. Halo D–Halo P tracings are 10 bipolar electrograms recorded from the distal (low lateral right atrium) to proximal (high right atrium) poles of the 20-pole Halo catheter positioned around the tricuspid valve annulus with the proximal electrode pair at the 1:00 o'clock position and the distal electrode pair at the 7:00 o'clock position. CSP: electrograms recorded from the coronary sinus catheter proximal electrode pair positioned at the ostium of the coronary sinus; HISP: electrograms recorded from the proximal electrode pair of the His bundle catheter; RF: electrograms recorded from the mapping and ablation catheter positioned with the distal electrode pair in the cavo-tricuspid isthmus. (Source: Adapted from Feld GK, Srivatsa U, Hoppe B, 2006[52]. Reproduced with permission from Elsevier, Copyright © 2006 Elsevier).

positioned fluoroscopically (Figure 7.3) across the CTI, with the distal ablation electrode near the tricuspid valve annulus in the right anterior oblique view, and midway between the septum and low right atrial free wall (in the 6 or 7 o'clock position) in the left anterior oblique (LAO) view. When appropriately positioned, the distal ablation electrode records an atrial-to-ventricular electrogram amplitude ratio of 1 : 2 to 1 : 4 (Figure 7.4a). For RFCA, the ablation catheter is gradually withdrawn a few millimeters at a time across the entire CTI, pausing for 30–60 seconds at each location, during a continuous or interrupted energy application. RFCA of the CTI may require several sequential 30–60 sec energy applications during a stepwise catheter pullback, or a prolonged energy application of up to 120 sec or more during a continuous catheter pullback. Radiofrequency energy application should be immediately interrupted when the catheter has reached the inferior vena cava, since ablation in the venous structures is known to cause significant pain.

Procedure endpoints for ablation of AFL

Ablation may be performed during AFL or sinus rhythm. If ablation is performed during AFL, the first endpoint is its termination (Figure 7.6). Despite termination of AFL, however, CTI conduction commonly persists. Following ablation, electrophysiologic testing should be performed by pacing at a cycle length of 600 msec (or greater, depending on the sinus cycle length) to determine if there is bidirectional CTI conduction block (Figures 7.7 and

7.8). Bidirectional CTI conduction block is confirmed by demonstrating a strictly cranial-to-caudal activation sequence in the contralateral right atrium during pacing from the coronary sinus ostium or low lateral right atrium, respectively,[34–36] and recording widely spaced double potentials (≥100 msec apart) along the ablation line during pacing lateral or medial to the line (Figure 7.9).[37,38] The presence of bidirectional CTI conduction block after ablation is associated with a significantly lower recurrence rate of AFL during long-term follow-up.[34–36,39] Pacing should be repeated at least 30–60 min after ablation to ensure that bidirectional CTI block persists, and burst pacing should be performed to ensure that AFL cannot be reinduced after ablation.[3,5–7,24–28,30–33,40] If CTI block is not achieved with either an 8–10 mm tip electrode catheter or a cooled-tip ablation catheter, crossing over to the alternative catheter or another energy source may be successful.[41]

Outcomes of radiofrequency catheter ablation of typical AFL

Early reports[3–6] on AFL ablation revealed recurrence rates up to 20–45% (Table 7.1). However, more contemporary studies have demonstrated acute and chronic success rates in excess of 95%. These improved results have been attributed to confirmation of bidirectional CTI conduction block as an endpoint for successful ablation of AFL.[24–33] Patients with difficult CTI anatomy due to a pouch or longer isthmus may have a higher incidence of recurrent CTI conduction in long-term follow-up.[42]

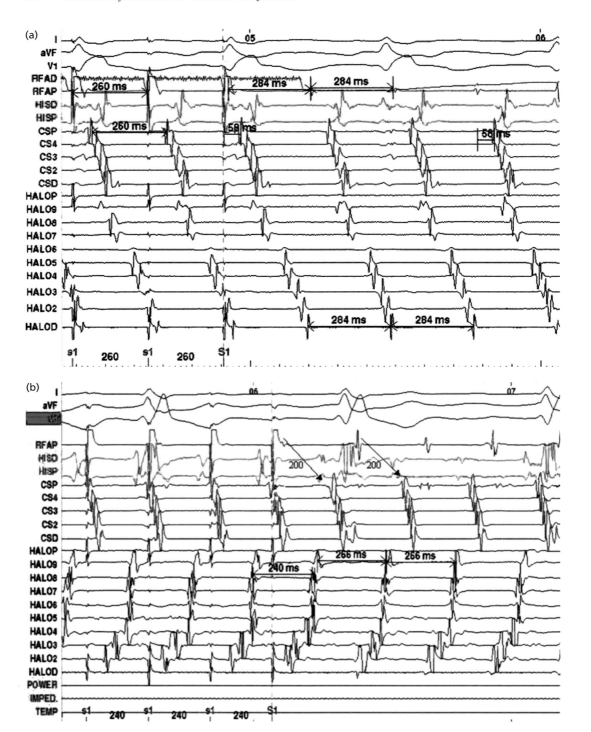

Figure 7.5. Endocardial electrograms from the RF, Halo, CS, and His bundle catheters, and surface ECG leads I, aVF, and V1, are shown, demonstrating concealed entrainment from an RF ablation catheter positioned in the cavo-tricuspid isthmus (CTI) in a patient with (a) typical AFL and (b) reverse typical AFL. Note that the tachycardia is accelerated to the pacing cycle length, the tachycardia continues upon termination of pacing, the first postpacing interval and the tachycardia cycle length are equal (284 vs. 284 and 266 vs. 266 msec) , the stimulus to proximal CS electrogram time and the local electrogram on the RF catheter to proximal CS electrogram time are the same (58 vs. 58 and 200 vs. 200 msec), and there is no change in activation sequence, endocardial electrograms, or surface P wave morphology. Halo D–Halo P are 10 bipolar electrograms recorded from the distal (low lateral right atrium) to proximal (high right atrium) poles of the 20-pole Halo catheter positioned around the tricuspid valve annulus with the proximal electrode pair at the 1 o'clock position and the distal electrode pair at the 7 o'clock position. CSP-D: electrograms recorded from the coronary sinus catheter proximal to distal electrode pairs, with the proximal pair positioned at the ostium of the coronary sinus; HISP&D: electrograms recorded from the proximal and distal electrode pair of the His bundle catheter; RFAP&D: electrograms recorded from the proximal and distal electrode pairs of the mapping and ablation catheter positioned in the CTI. (Source: Adapted from Feld GK, Srivatsa U, Hoppe B, 2006[52]. Reproduced with permission from Elsevier, Copyright © 2006 Elsevier).

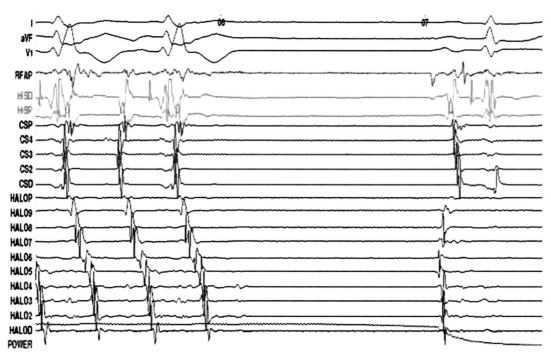

Figure 7.6. Surface electrocardiogram (ECG) and endocardial electrogram recordings during ablation of the cavo-tricuspid isthmus (CTI) at the time of termination of typical atrial flutter (AFL). Note the abrupt termination of AFL, which occurred in this patient as the ablation catheter reached the Eustachian ridge, followed by restoration of normal sinus rhythm. I, aVF, and V1: surface ECG leads; RFAP: proximal ablation electrogram; Hisp&d: proximal and distal His bundle electrograms; CSd-p: distal to proximal coronary sinus electrograms; Halo d–p: distal to proximal Halo catheter electrograms; Imped: impedance; Temp: temperature. (Source: Adapted from Feld GK, Birgersdotter-Green U, Narayan S, 2007[8]. Reproduced with permission from John Wiley and Sons Ltd).

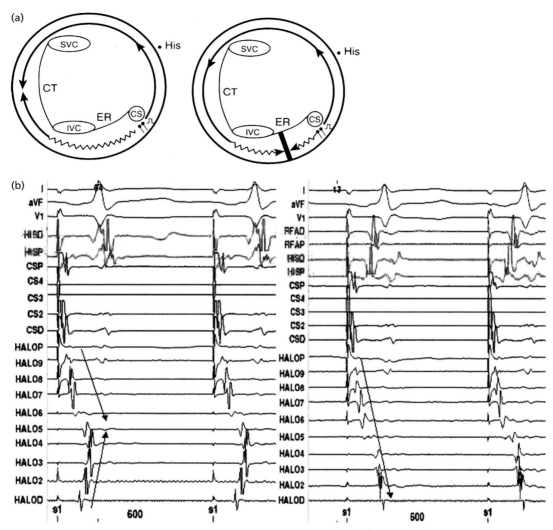

Figure 7.7. (a) A schematic diagram of the expected right atrial activation sequence during pacing in sinus rhythm from the coronary sinus (CS) ostium before (left panel) and after (right panel) ablation of the cavo-tricuspid isthmus (CTI). Prior to ablation, the activation pattern during CS pacing is caudal to cranial in the interatrial septum and low right atrium, with collision of the septal and right atrial wavefronts in the midlateral right atrium. Following ablation, the activation pattern during coronary sinus pacing is still caudal to cranial in the interatrial septum, but the lateral right atrium is now activated in a strictly cranial-to-caudal pattern (i.e., counterclockwise), indicating complete clockwise conduction block in the CTI. CT: crista terminalis; ER: Eustachian ridge; His: His bundle; IVC: inferior vena cava; SVC: superior vena cava. (b) Surface electrocardiogram (ECG) and right atrial endocardial electrograms recorded during pacing in sinus rhythm from the CS ostium before (left panel) and after (right panel) ablation of the CTI. Tracings include surface ECG leads I, aVF, and V1, and endocardial electrograms from the proximal coronary sinus (CSP), His bundle (HIS), tricuspid valve annulus at the 1:00 o'clock position (HaloP) to the 7:00 o'clock position (HaloD), and high right atrium (HRA or RFA). Prior to ablation during CS pacing, there is collision of the cranial and caudal right atrial wavefronts in the midlateral right atrium (HALO5). Following ablation, the lateral right atrium is activated in a strictly cranial-to-caudal pattern (i.e., counterclockwise), indicating complete medial-to-lateral conduction block in the CTI. (Source: Adapted from Feld GK, Srivatsa U, Hoppe B, 2006[52]. Reproduced with permission from Elsevier, Copyright © 2006 Elsevier).

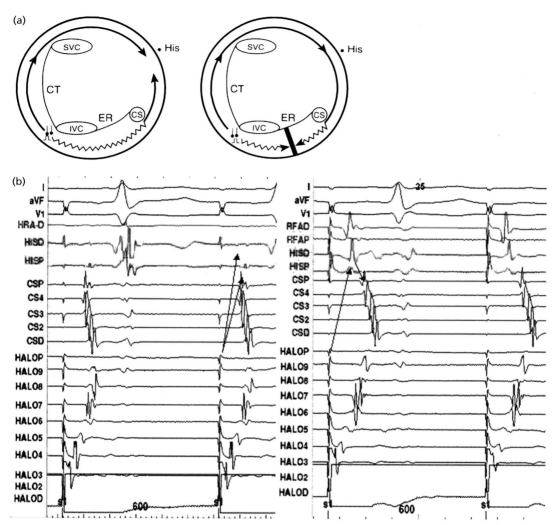

Figure 7.8. (a) Schematic diagrams of the expected right atrial activation sequence during pacing in sinus rhythm from the low lateral right atrium before (left panel) and after (right panel) ablation of the cavo-tricuspid isthmus (CTI). Prior to ablation, the activation pattern during coronary sinus (CS) pacing is caudal to cranial in the right atrial free wall, with collision of the cranial and caudal wavefronts in the midseptum, and with simultaneous activation at the His bundle (HISP) and proximal coronary sinus (CSP). Following ablation, the activation pattern during low lateral right atrial sinus pacing is still caudal to cranial in the right atrial free wall, but the septum is now activated in a strictly cranial-to-caudal pattern (i.e., clockwise), indicating complete lateral-to-medial conduction block in the CTI. CT: crista terminalis, ER: Eustachian ridge, His: His bundle, SVC: superior vena cava, IVC: inferior vena cava. (b) Surface electrocardiogram (ECG) and right atrial endocardial electrograms during pacing in sinus rhythm from the low lateral right atrium before (left panel) and after (right panel) ablation of the CTI. Tracings include surface ECG leads I, aVF and V1, and endocardial electrograms from the proximal coronary sinus (CSP), His bundle (HIS), tricuspid valve annulus at the 1:00 o'clock position (HaloP) to the 7:00 o'clock position (HaloD), and high right atrium (HRA or RFA). Prior to ablation during low lateral right atrial pacing, there is collision of the cranial and caudal right atrial wavefronts in the midseptum (HIS and CSP). Following ablation, the septum is activated in a strictly cranial-to-caudal pattern (i.e., clockwise), indicating complete lateral-to-medial conduction block in the CTI. (Source: Adapted from Feld GK, Srivatsa U, Hoppe B, 2006[52]. Reproduced with permission from Elsevier, Copyright © 2006 Elsevier).

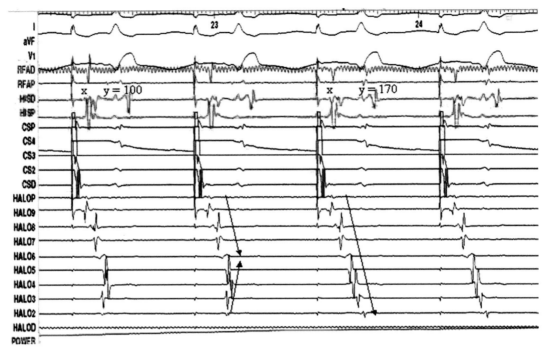

Figure 7.9. Surface electrocardiogram (ECG) leads I, aVF, and V1, and endocardial electrograms from the coronary sinus, His bundle, Halo, mapping and ablation (RF), and right ventricular catheters during radiofrequency catheter ablation of the cavo-tricuspid isthmus (CTI) during pacing from the coronary sinus ostium. Note the change in activation sequence in the lateral right atrium on the Halo catheter from bidirectional to unidirectional, indicating the development of clockwise block in the CTI. This was associated with development of widely spaced (170 msec) double potentials (x and y) on the RF catheter along the ablation line, confirming medial-to-lateral conduction block. All abbreviations are the same as in the other figures of this chapter. (Source: Adapted from Feld GK, Birgersdotter-Green U, Narayan S, 2007[8]. Reproduced with permission from John Wiley and Sons Ltd).

Furthermore, randomized studies of irrigated versus large-tip radiofrequency ablation catheters suggest a slightly higher success rate with the externally cooled ablation catheters, compared to internally cooled ablation catheters or large-tip ablation catheters.[27,28,30,33,40]

RFCA for typical AFL is relatively safe, but serious complications can occur, including AV block, cardiac perforation and tamponade, and thromboembolic events including pulmonary embolism and stroke. However, in recent large-scale studies, including those using large-tip catheters and high-power generators, major complications have been observed in only 2.5–3.0% of patients.[32,33,40]

Cryocatheter ablation of typical AFL

The development of new energy sources for ablation of AFL has been driven in part by the disadvantages of RFCA, including pain produced by RFCA, the risk of coagulum formation and embolization, tissue charring, and subendocardial steam pops resulting in perforation. Several clinical and pre-clinical studies have recently been published on the use of catheter cryoablation of AFL.[43–51] Recent studies have demonstrated that catheter cryoablation of typical AFL can be achieved with short- and long-term results similar to, or slightly below, those achieved with RFCA.[43–51] The potential advantages

Table 7.1. Success rates for radiofrequency catheter ablation of atrial flutter

Author (year)	N	Electrode length	% acute success	Follow-up (months)	% chronic success
Feld et al. (1992)[5]	16	4	100	4 ± 2	83
Cosio et al. (1993)[6]	9	4	100	2–18	56
Kirkorian et al. (1994)[25]	22	4	86	8 ± 13	84
Fischer et al. (1995)[24]	80	4	73	20 ± 8	81
Poty et al. (1995)[35]	12	6/8	100	9 ± 3	92
Schwartzman et al. (1996)[36]	35	8	100	1–21	92
Cauchemez et al. (1996)[39]	20	4	100	8 ± 2	80
Tsai et al. (1999)[31]	50	8	92	10 ± 5	100
Atiga et al. (2002)[30]	59	4 vs. cooled	88	13 ± 4	93
Scavee et al. (2004)[28]	80	8 vs. cooled	80	15	98
Feld et al. (2004)[32]	169	8 or 10	93	6	97
Calkins et al. (2004)[40]	150	8	88	6	87
Ventura et al. (2004)[33]	130	8 vs. cooled	100	14 ± 2	98

N: number of patients studied; % acute success: termination of atrial flutter during ablation and/or demonstration of isthmus block following ablation; % chronic success: % of patients in whom type 1 atrial flutter did not recur during follow-up. Acute and chronic success rates are reported as overall results in randomized or comparison studies.

of cryoablation over RFCA, however, include less pain associated with ablation,[44,51] and the lack of tissue charring or coagulum formation. See Video Clip 7.1.

The technical approach to catheter cryoablation is essentially identical to that described here for RFCA, with the exception that during each ablation freeze the cryoablation catheter cannot be moved as it becomes frozen to the tissue within seconds of onset of each ablation, and there is loss of endocardial electrogram recordings due to ice ball formation around the ablation electrode during each ablation. Target temperatures for catheter cryoablation are typically −80 to −90 °C, with freeze durations at each location up to 4 min (e.g., a single ablation up to 4 min or double 2 min freezes). The cryoablation catheter can be moved only between freezes, after thawing of the ice ball, which typically occurs within 30–60 sec after termination of freezing. Since it is preferable to overlap freezes, the cryoablation catheter should not be withdrawn across the CTI more than the length of the ablation electrode between each freeze. The endpoints for catheter cryoablation of the CTI are identical to those with RFCA, including termination of AFL if present at onset of electrophysiologic study, and creation of

bidirectional CTI conduction block for a minimum duration of 30 min after ablation.

In the largest study of catheter cryoablation of AFL published to date,[50] catheter cryoablation was performed using a 10 Fr catheter with a 6.5 mm metal tip and a cryogenerator capable of producing nadir temperatures of −90 °C (CryoCor, Inc., CA, United States) in 160 patients with CTI-dependent AFL. There were 122 men and 38 women, whose mean age was 63.1 ± 9.3 years, and in whom the mean left ventricular ejection fraction was 54.6 ± 10.4%. Of these patients, 94 (58.8%) also had a history of atrial fibrillation. All patients underwent right atrial (RA) activation mapping and pacing at the CTI to demonstrate concealed entrainment and confirm the CTI dependence of AFL.

Cryoablation of the CTI was performed with multiple freezes (average freeze time 2.3 ± 0.5 min, range 2–5 min) from the tricuspid valve annulus, through the CTI, to the Eustachian ridge, until bidirectional block was demonstrated during pacing from the low lateral RA and coronary sinus, respectively. A catheter cryoablation freeze was considered effective if the catheter position was stable at the targeted location, a nadir temperature near −90 °C was reached during ablation, and the freeze duration was at least 2 min. Acute procedural success was defined as CTI block persisting 30 min after ablation. Immediate repeat cryoablation was performed if CTI conduction recurred during the waiting period. If bidirectional CTI block could not be achieved with catheter cryoablation, the CTI could be ablated with an approved RFCA device, at which point the patient was considered a catheter cryoablation failure and discharged from the study.

Patients were evaluated at 1, 3, and 6 months and underwent once-weekly and symptomatic-event monitoring. Long-term success was defined as absence of symptomatic or monitored AFL during follow-up. Acute success with bidirectional CTI block was achieved in 140 (87.5%) of 160 patients. Total procedure time was 200 ± 71 minutes, ablation time (including a 30 min waiting period after ablation) 139 ± 62 minutes, and fluoroscopy time 35 ± 26 minutes. An average of 20.5 ± 11.3 freezes, for a total ablation time of 47.4 ± 24.3 minutes, was required to achieve bidi-

rectional CTI block, with average and nadir temperatures of −81.5 ± 3.7 °C and −85.6 ± 3.6 °C, respectively.

Of 132 patients with acute efficacy who completed 6 months of follow-up, 8 (6%) were lost to follow-up or were noncompliant with event recordings. Using survival analysis, 106 (80.3%) remained free of AFL on strict analysis of event recordings only (Figure 7.10), and 119 (90.2%) remained clinically free of AFL (Figure 7.11).

Of the 160 patients treated, 9 (5.6%) had serious adverse events (one per patient) within 7 days post ablation. These serious adverse events were atrial fibrillation in one, a groin hematoma in one, cardiac tamponade in one, dizziness in one, acute respiratory failure in one, AFL in one, sick sinus syndrome in two, and complete AV block in one. The data safety and monitoring board characterized only four (2.50%) serious adverse events as device and/or procedure related, specifically groin hematoma in one, cardiac tamponade 6 days post ablation in

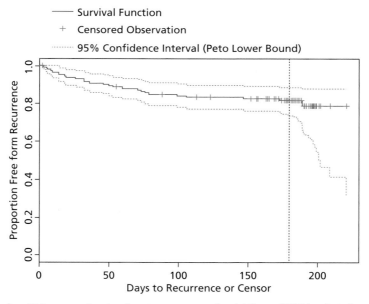

Figure 7.10. Kaplan–Meier curve showing days to recurrence of atrial flutter (AFL) by clinical analysis of symptomatic AFL recurrence. Patients were censored if they were lost to follow-up or were noncompliant with event monitoring. The solid line represents survival function, the dashed line represents the 95% confidence interval, and hash marks represent points of censor. (Source: Feld GK, Daubert JP, Weiss R, Miles WM, and Pelkey W, 2008[50]. Reproduced with permission from Elsevier. Copyright © 2008, Elsevier).

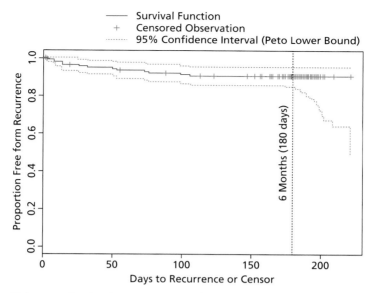

Figure 7.11. Kaplan–Meier curve showing days to recurrence of AFL documented by event monitor. Patients were censored if they were lost to follow-up or were noncompliant with event monitoring. The solid line represents survival function, the dashed line represents the 95% confidence interval, and hash marks represent points of censoring. (Source: Feld GK, Daubert JP, Weiss R, Miles WM, and Pelkey W, 2008[50]. Reproduced with permission from Elsevier. Copyright © 2008, Elsevier).

one, acute respiratory failure in one, and complete AV block requiring pacemaker implantation in one. The single instance of AV block resulted from extensive medial CTI ablation and was permanent. All these adverse events, except for the AV block, resolved by the end of the study.

In a more recent, prospective, randomized study of catheter cryoablation versus RFCA for typical AFL,[51] a total of 191 patients were randomized to RFCA or catheter cryoablation of the CTI using an 8 mm tip catheter in both groups (catheter cryoablation was performed with the Freezor MAX, Cryo-Cath, Inc., Quebec, Canada). In all patients, bidirectional conduction block of the CTI was defined as the ablation endpoint. The primary endpoint of the study was lack of persistence of bidirectional CTI conduction block and/or ECG-documented recurrence of typical AFL within 3-month follow-up. The acute success rates were 91% (83/91) in the radiofrequency group and 89% (80/90) in the catheter cryoablation group (p = NS). However, the procedure time was significantly longer in the catheter cryoablation group compared

to the RFCA group (120 versus 99 min, $p < .01$). Symptomatic typical AFL recurred during follow-up in seven patients in the catheter cryoablation group, but in none in the RFCA group. Invasive electrophysiologic study was performed after 3-month follow-up in 60 patients in the RFCA group and 64 patients in the catheter cryoablation group. Persistent bidirectional CTI conduction block was confirmed in 85% of the RFCA group versus 65.6% of the catheter cryoablation group. The primary endpoint was thus achieved in 15% of patients in the RFCA group, but in 34.4% of patients in the catheter cryoablation group ($p = .014$). Pain perception (defined using a visual analog pain scale with a range of 0–100), a secondary endpoint during ablation, was significant lower in the catheter cryoablation group compared to the RFCA group (0 versus 60, $p < .001$).

In this study, there were five patients who developed adverse events (2.5%), with one patient developing complete AV block and one developing a stroke, in the catheter cryoablation group.[51] The remaining three patients developed vascular complications, including two groin hematomas and one arterial pseudoaneurysm.

Summary

Radiofrequency catheter ablation has become a first-line treatment for AFL, due in combination to its cost-effectiveness, its high acute and chronic success rates, and its low complication rates. The use of large-tip (i.e., 8–10 mm) or irrigated ablation catheters is recommended for optimal success. Catheter cryoablation has also been shown to be effective for treatment of typical AFL, producing acute bidirectional CTI block rates similar to those achieved with RFCA. However, long-term suppression rates of AFL may be slightly less with catheter cryoablation compared to RFCA, due to recovery of CTI conduction. The reason for higher rates of recovery of CTI conduction with catheter cryoablation compared to RFCA is unclear, but may be due to less tissue structural damage produced during ablation. Although catheter cryoablation may take somewhat longer to perform than RFCA of the CTI, catheter cryoablation may be accomplished with less perceived pain during ablation compared to RFCA. Complication rates with catheter cryoablation are similar to those seen during RFCA.

 Interactive Case Studies related to this chapter can be found at this book's companion website, at
www.chancryoablation.com

References

1. Saoudi N, Cosio F, Waldo A, et al. Classification of atrial flutter and regular atrial tachycardia according to electrophysiologic mechanism and anatomic bases: a statement from a joint expert group from the Working Group of Arrhythmias of the European Society of Cardiology and the North American Society of Pacing and Electrophysiology. J Cardiovasc Electrophysiol. 2001;12:852–66.

2. Olshansky B, Okumura K, Hess PG, et al. Demonstration of an area of slow conduction in human atrial flutter. J Am Coll Cardiol. 1990;16:1639–48.

3. Lesh MD, Van Hare GF, Epstein LM, et al. Radiofrequency catheter ablation of atrial arrhythmias. Results and mechanisms. Circulation. 1994;89:1074–89.

4. Cosio FG, Goicolea A, Lopez-Gil M, et al. Atrial endocardial mapping in the rare form of atrial flutter. Am J Cardiol. 1990;66:715–20.

5. Feld GK, Fleck RP, Chen PS, et al. Radiofrequency catheter ablation for the treatment of human type 1 atrial flutter. Identification of a critical zone in the reentrant circuit by endocardial mapping techniques. Circulation. 1992;86:1233–40.

6. Cosio FG, Lopez-Gil M, Goicolea A, et al. Radiofrequency ablation of the inferior vena cava-tricuspid valve isthmus in common atrial flutter. Am J Cardiol. 1993;71:705–9.

7. Tai CT, Chen SA, Chiang CE, et al. Electrophysiologic characteristics and radiofrequency catheter ablation in patients with clockwise atrial flutter. J Cardiovasc Electrophysiol. 1997;8:24–34.

8. Feld GK, Mollerus M, Birgersdotter-Green U, et al. Conduction velocity in the tricuspid valve-inferior vena cava isthmus is slower in patients with type I atrial flutter compared to those without a history of atrial flutter. J Cardiovasc Electrophysiol. 1997;8:1338–48.

9. Kinder C, Kall J, Kopp D, et al. Conduction properties of the inferior vena cava-tricuspid annular isthmus in patients with typical atrial flutter. J Cardiovasc Electrophysiol. 1997;8:727–37.

10. Da Costa A, Mourot S, Romeyer-Bouchard C, et al. Anatomic and electrophysiological differences between chronic and paroxysmal forms of common atrial flutter and comparison with controls. Pacing Clin Electrophysiol. 2004;27:1202–11.

11. Kalman JM, Olgin JE, Saxon LA, et al. Activation and entrainment mapping defines the tricuspid annulus as the anterior barrier in typical atrial flutter. Circulation. 1996;94:398–406.

12. Olgin JE, Kalman JM, Lesh MD. Conduction barriers in human atrial flutter: correlation of electrophysiology and anatomy. J Cardiovasc Electrophysiol. 1996;7:1112–26.

13. Olgin JE, Kalman JM, Fitzpatrick AP, et al. Role of right atrial endocardial structures as barriers to conduction during human type I atrial flutter. Activation and entrainment mapping guided by intracardiac echocardiography. Circulation. 1995;92:1839–48.

14. Tai CT, Huang JL, Lee PC, et al. High-resolution mapping around the crista terminalis during typical atrial flutter: new insights into mechanisms. J Cardiovasc Electrophysiol. 2004;15:406–14.

15. Spach MS, Dolber PC, Heidlage JF. Influence of the passive anisotropic properties on directional differences in propagation following modification of the sodium conductance in human atrial muscle. A

model of reentry based on anisotropic discontinuous propagation. Circ Res. 1988;62:811–32.

16. Spach MS, Miller WT, III, Dolber PC, *et al.* The functional role of structural complexities in the propagation of depolarization in the atrium of the dog. Cardiac conduction disturbances due to discontinuities of effective axial resistivity. Circ Res. 1982;50: 175–91.

17. Olgin JE, Kalman JM, Saxon LA, *et al.* Mechanism of initiation of atrial flutter in humans: site of unidirectional block and direction of rotation. J Am Coll Cardiol. 1997;29:376–84.

18. Suzuki F, Toshida N, Nawata H, *et al.* Coronary sinus pacing initiates counterclockwise atrial flutter while pacing from the low lateral right atrium initiates clockwise atrial flutter. Analysis of episodes of direct initiation of atrial flutter. J Electrocardiol. 1998;31: 345–61.

19. Feld GK, Shahandeh-Rad F. Activation patterns in experimental canine atrial flutter produced by right atrial crush injury. J Am Coll Cardiol. 1992;20: 441–51.

20. Haissaguerre M, Sanders P, Hocini M, *et al.* Pulmonary veins in the substrate for atrial fibrillation: the "venous wave" hypothesis. J Am Coll Cardiol. 2004; 43:2290–2.

21. Oshikawa N, Watanabe I, Masaki R, *et al.* Relationship between polarity of the flutter wave in the surface ECG and endocardial atrial activation sequence in patients with typical counterclockwise and clockwise atrial flutter. J Interv Card Electrophysiol. 2002;7: 215–23.

22. Okumura K, Plumb VJ, Page PL, *et al.* Atrial activation sequence during atrial flutter in the canine pericarditis model and its effects on the polarity of the flutter wave in the electrocardiogram. J Am Coll Cardiol. 1991;17:509–18.

23. Chugh A, Latchamsetty R, Oral H, *et al.* Characteristics of cavotricuspid isthmus-dependent atrial flutter after left atrial ablation of atrial fibrillation. Circulation. 2006;113:609–15.

24. Fischer B, Haissaguerre M, Garrigues S, *et al.* Radiofrequency catheter ablation of common atrial flutter in 80 patients. J Am Coll Cardiol. 1995;25: 1365–72.

25. Kirkorian G, Moncada E, Chevalier P, *et al.* Radiofrequency ablation of atrial flutter. Efficacy of an anatomically guided approach. Circulation. 1994;90: 2804–14.

26. Calkins H, Leon AR, Deam AG, *et al.* Catheter ablation of atrial flutter using radiofrequency energy. Am J Cardiol. 1994;73:353–6.

27. Jais P, Haissaguerre M, Shah DC, *et al.* Successful irrigated-tip catheter ablation of atrial flutter resist-

ant to conventional radiofrequency ablation. Circulation. 1998;98:835–8.

28. Scavee C, Jais P, Hsu LF, *et al.* Prospective randomised comparison of irrigated-tip and large-tip catheter ablation of cavotricuspid isthmus-dependent atrial flutter. Eur Heart J. 2004;25:963–9.

29. Calkins H. Catheter ablation of atrial flutter: do outcomes of catheter ablation with "large-tip" versus "cooled-tip" catheters really differ? J Cardiovasc Electrophysiol. 2004;15:1131–2.

30. Atiga WL, Worley SJ, Hummel J, *et al.* Prospective randomized comparison of cooled radiofrequency versus standard radiofrequency energy for ablation of typical atrial flutter. Pacing Clin Electrophysiol. 2002;25:1172–8.

31. Tsai CF, Tai CT, Yu WC, *et al.* Is 8-mm more effective than 4-mm tip electrode catheter for ablation of typical atrial flutter? Circulation. 1999;100: 768–71.

32. Feld G, Wharton M, Plumb V, *et al.* Radiofrequency catheter ablation of type 1 atrial flutter using large-tip 8- or 10-mm electrode catheters and a high-output radiofrequency energy generator: results of a multicenter safety and efficacy study. J Am Coll Cardiol. 2004;43:1466–72.

33. Ventura R, Klemm H, Lutomsky B, *et al.* Pattern of isthmus conduction recovery using open cooled and solid large-tip catheters for radiofrequency ablation of typical atrial flutter. J Cardiovasc Electrophysiol. 2004;15:1126–30.

34. Mangat I, Tschopp DR, Jr., Yang Y, *et al.* Optimizing the detection of bidirectional block across the flutter isthmus for patients with typical isthmus-dependent atrial flutter. Am J Cardiol. 2003;91:559–64.

35. Poty H, Saoudi N, Abdel Aziz A, *et al.* Radiofrequency catheter ablation of type 1 atrial flutter. Prediction of late success by electrophysiological criteria. Circulation. 1995;92:1389–92.

36. Schwartzman D, Callans DJ, Gottlieb CD, *et al.* Conduction block in the inferior vena caval-tricuspid valve isthmus: association with outcome of radiofrequency ablation of type I atrial flutter. J Am Coll Cardiol. 1996;28:1519–31.

37. Tada H, Oral H, Sticherling C, *et al.* Double potentials along the ablation line as a guide to radiofrequency ablation of typical atrial flutter. J Am Coll Cardiol. 2001;38:750–5.

38. Tai CT, Haque A, Lin YK, *et al.* Double potential interval and transisthmus conduction time for prediction of cavotricuspid isthmus block after ablation of typical atrial flutter. J Interv Card Electrophysiol. 2002;7:77–82.

39. Cauchemez B, Haissaguerre M, Fischer B, *et al.* Electrophysiological effects of catheter ablation of inferior

vena cava-tricuspid annulus isthmus in common atrial flutter. Circulation. 1996;93:284–94.

40. Calkins H, Canby R, Weiss R, *et al*. Results of catheter ablation of typical atrial flutter. Am J Cardiol. 2004;94:437–42.

41. Ilg KJ, Kuhne M, Crawford T, *et al*. Randomized comparison of cavotricuspid isthmus ablation for atrial flutter using an open irrigation-tip versus a large-tip radiofrequency ablation catheter. J Cardiovasc Electrophysiol. 2011;22:1007–12.

42. Lo LW, Tai CT, Lin YJ, *et al*. Characteristics of the cavotricuspid isthmus in predicting recurrent conduction in the long-term follow-up. J Cardiovasc Electrophysiol. 2009;20:39–43.

43. Manusama R, Timmermans C, Limon F, *et al*. Catheter-based cryoablation permanently cures patients with common atrial flutter. Circulation. 2004;109:1636–9.

44. Timmermans C, Ayers GM, Crijns HJ, *et al*. Randomized study comparing radiofrequency ablation with cryoablation for the treatment of atrial flutter with emphasis on pain perception. Circulation. 2003; 107:1250–2.

45. Daubert JP, Hoyt RH, John R, *et al*. Performance of a new cardiac cryoablation system in the treatment of cavotricuspid valve isthmus-dependent atrial flutter. Pacing Clin Electrophysiol. 2005;28:S142–5.

46. Montenero AS, Bruno N, Antonelli A, *et al*. Long-term efficacy of cryo catheter ablation for the treatment of atrial flutter: results from a repeat electrophysiologic study. J Am Coll Cardiol. 2005;45:573–80.

47. Montenero AS, Bruno N, Antonelli A, *et al*. Comparison between a 7 French 6 mm tip cryothermal catheter and a 9 French 8 mm tip cryothermal catheter for cryoablation treatment of common atrial flutter. J Interv Card Electrophysiol. 2005;13:59–69.

48. Montenero AS, Bruno N, Zumbo F, *et al*. Cryothermal ablation treatment of atrial flutter-experience with a new 9 French 8-mm-tip catheter. J Interv Card Electrophysiol. 2005;12:45–54.

49. Kuniss M, Kurzidim K, Greiss H, *et al*. Acute success and persistence of bidirectional conduction block in the cavotricuspid isthmus one month post cryocatheter ablation of common atrial flutter. Pacing Clin Electrophysiol. 2006;29:146–52.

50. Feld GK, Daubert JP, Weiss R, *et al*. Acute and long-term efficacy and safety of catheter cryoablation of the cavotricuspid isthmus for treatment of type 1 atrial flutter. Heart Rhythm. 2008;5:1009–14.

51. Kuniss M, Vogtmann T, Ventura R, *et al*. Prospective randomized comparison of durability of bidirectional conduction block in the cavotricuspid isthmus in patients after ablation of common atrial flutter using cryothermy and radiofrequency energy: the CRYOTIP study. Heart Rhythm. 2009;6:1699–705.

52. Feld GK, Srivatsa U, Hoppe B. Ablation of isthmus dependent atrial flutters. In: Huang SS, Wood MA, editors. Catheter ablation of cardiac arrhythmias. Philadelphia: Elsevier; 2006. p. 195–218.

CHAPTER 8

Catheter Cryoablation for the Treatment of Accessory Pathways

Ngai-Yin Chan

Princess Margaret Hospital, Hong Kong, China

Catheter ablation with radiofrequency (RF) energy is now a well-accepted first-line therapeutic option in accessory pathway (AP)–mediated arrhythmias. Depending on symptoms, it belongs to either the Class I or Class IIa indication for catheter ablation.[1] Radiofrequency catheter ablation (RFCA) has been reputed for its high acute procedural success rate and low rates of complications and recurrences in the treatment of APs.[2–10] However, a number of limitations of RF energy exist. RFCA of septal APs remains challenging with a lower acute procedural success, higher recurrence rate, and, most importantly, higher risk of inadvertent atrioventricular block (AVB). Collateral damage to coronary arteries and autonomic nerves has also been recognized as a potential complication of using RF energy in ablating APs.

In this chapter, the data on RF catheter ablation of APs will be reviewed with special emphasis on its limitations. The use of an alternative source of energy, cryothermy, in the treatment of APs will be discussed in detail, including its potential advantages, practical application, current data, and limitations.

Performance of RFCA of APs

In general, RFCA of APs enjoys a high acute procedural success rate, and low complication and recurrence rates. However, the performance of this energy source is in fact dependent on the location of the AP (Table 8.1). The overall acute procedural success rate varies from 80% to 99%. In the most recent series reported by Dagres et al.[11] and Kobza et al.,[12] it was 92 and 95%, respectively. The acute procedural success rates for both right free wall (RFW) and septal AP appeared lower than those of the left free wall (LFW) pathways. Moreover, the recurrence rate of RFW and septal APs are significantly higher than those of the LFW pathways. Kobza et al.[12] reported a 17% and 19% recurrence rate for RFW and septal pathways after RFCA, whereas the recurrence rate for LFW APs was only 5%. Inadvertent permanent AVB complicating RFCA is rare for both LFW and RFW APs. However, it happened in 2–3% of patients with septal pathways ablated with the RF energy source.

Table 8.1. Performance of radiofrequency catheter ablation in the treatment of accessory pathways

Authors	All				Left free wall pathways				Right free wall pathways				Septal pathways			
	N	APS (%)	AVB (%)	R (%)	N	APS (%)	AVB (%)	R (%)	N	APS (%)	AVB (%)	R (%)	N	APS (%)	AVB (%)	R (%)
Jackman (1991)[2]	166	164 (99)	0 (0.6)	15 (9)	105	105 (100)	0	5 (5)	14	14 (100)	0	2 (14)	56	53 (95)	1 (2)	8 (9)
Lesh* (1992)[5]	109	98 (90)	0	8 (9)	45	44 (98)	0	N/A	21	17 (80)	0	N/A	43	36 (84)	0	N/A
Swartz* (1993)[7]	122	116 (95)	1 (0.8)	10 (9)	76	74 (97)	0	5 (7)	12	8 (67)	0	2 (17)	34	N/A	1 (3)	3 (9)
Kay* (1993)[6]	384	367 (96)	0	19 (5)	187	186 (99)	0	4 (2)	62	57 (92)	0	5 (9)	131	122 (93)	0	N/A
Scheinmann* (1995)[9]	5427	4889 (90)	9 (0.2)	N/A	3096	2879 (93)	N/A	N/A	885	752 (85)	N/A	N/A	1446	1258 (87)	N/A	N/A
Calkins (1999)[10]	500	398 (80)	5 (1)	31 (8)	270	224 (82)	1 (0.3)	7 (3)	92	66 (72)	0	9 (14)	138	108 (78)	4 (3)	15 (14)
Dagres (2003)[11]	519	476 (92)	N/A	50 (10)	N/A	N/A	N/A	N/A	N/A	N/A	N/A	N/A	N/A	N/A	N/A	N/A
Kobza (2005)[12]	318	302 (95)	2 (0.6)	32 (10)	181	178 (98)	0	9 (5)	36	35 (97)	0	6 (17)	101	89 (88)	2 (2)	17 (19)

APS: acute procedural success; AVB: permanent atrioventricular block; N/A: not available; R: recurrence.

*The numbers refer to accessory pathways instead of patients.

Uncommon complications of RFCA for APs

Some uncommon complications of RFCA for APs have been described. These include coronary artery spasm and injury,[13–17] autonomic nerve injury,[18–21] and inadvertent AVB during ablation of nonseptal APs.[22]

Coronary artery spasm and injury have been reported in both adults and children. Coronary artery spasm or even occlusion may occur if RF energy is delivered in close proximity to it. Left circumflex artery injury may occur during RF ablation of LFW APs.[14] Right coronary artery injury has been reported after ablation of RFW and posteroseptal APs.[15,16] Interestingly, occlusion of the left anterior descending artery has also been observed days after ablation of a LFW pathway.[17] Thrombus formation at the ablation site with subsequent coronary embolism may be the possible mechanism. Schneider et al. identified acute coronary artery narrowing in 2 out of 117 pediatric patients with RFCA for APs.[13] Both patients had posteroseptal pathways.

Persistent inappropriate sinus tachycardia and atrial arrhythmias were known to complicate RFCA treatment for supraventricular tachycardias.[23–27] The most likely mechanism is believed to be a disturbance of the sympathovagal balance after RFCA of some endocardial sites. Psychari et al. has shown efferent cardiac sympathetic denervation as evidenced by I-123 metaiodobenzylguanidine map defects in patients receiving RFCA for atrioventricular nodal reentrant tachycardia (AVNRT) and posteroseptal pathways, but not LFW APs.[28] At the same time, there was attenuation in both high- and low-frequency components of heart rate variability in patients with ablation of posteroseptal pathways. In patients with ablation for AVNRT, only the low-frequency component of heart rate variability was diminished. Attenuation of high- and low-frequency components in the frequency domain analysis of heart rate variability suggests decrease in parasympathetic and sympathetic activity, respectively. In contrast, Jinbo et al. demonstrated that only the high-frequency (but not low-frequency) component of heart rate variability was diminished in patients receiving RFCA for AVNRT and septal APs.[29] Emkanjoo et al. found no change in heart rate variability one month after ablation in patients with

AVNRT or APs in different locations. However, this may just indicate recovery of autonomic denervation one month after the injury.[20] The exact cause for the uncommon complication of persistent inappropriate sinus tachycardia thus remains controversial. The bulk of evidence seems to suggest damage to both parasympathetic and sympathetic components of the cardiac autonomic nervous system during RFCA in the anterior, middle, and posterior regions of the low interatrial septum.

The risk of AVB is relatively high during RFCA of septal APs. However, this complication has also been reported for LFW APs.[4,30–32] Calkins et al. reported an incidence of 1 in 270 in complete AVB complicating RFCA of LFW APs.[4] Potential mechanisms, including trauma to the atrioventricular (AV) node during catheter entry into the left ventricle, compression of the AV node by the catheter shaft, and anomaly of the AV node, have been postulated.

Potential advantages of using cryoablation instead of RFCA in the treatment of APs

In contrast with the RFCA lesion, which is more destructive and produces a diffuse area of hemorrhage and necrosis with thrombus formation, the cryolesion is characterized by disruption of membranous organelles with preservation of myocardial architecture.[33] It has been shown that after cryoablation, the endothelial layer remained intact, and thrombus formation was uncommon compared to RFCA.[34] With these favorable lesion characteristics, collateral damage during AP ablation (e.g. coronary artery injury) may be reduced with cryoablation. In an animal study, cryoablation inside the coronary sinus at locations within 2 mm of a coronary artery resulted in a transmural lesion similar to that of RFCA, but the risk of coronary artery stenosis is significantly lower with the former.[35,36]

The properties of producing, in general, a smaller lesion compared to those of RFCA, cryomapping, and cryoadhesion make cryothermy a more accurate energy source in creating a myocardial lesion. Although the lesion size of cryoablation is governed by multiple factors, it is in general smaller than that created by RF.[37] The capability of producing a reversible electrophysiological effect at a tissue temperature of $-30\,°C$ is termed *cryomapping*. If the reversible electrophysiological effect is regarded as desirable, a permanent lesion can be created by lowering the tissue temperature further to −75 °C. In animal studies, cryothermy of −30 °C delivered to the AV node by a catheter-based system resulted in a reversible modification of the AV node conduction without significant tissue damage.[38,39] Cryoadhesion occurs when the tissue temperature approaches 0 °C with ice formation. To prevent the complication of inadvertent AVB, these special properties of cryoablation make it the preferred energy source in treating septal APs.

Procedural techniques of cryoablation for accessory pathways

See Video Clip 8.1.

Baseline electrophysiology study

The basic setup for diagnostic electrophysiology study is similar to that of RFCA, with four electrode catheters positioned to the right atrium, His bundle, coronary sinus, and right ventricular apex, respectively. In case of a right free wall AP, a steerable decapolar catheter is positioned around the tricuspid valve annulus. The intracardiac activation pattern during both sinus rhythm and ventricular pacing is analyzed for localization of a manifested or concealed AP. Incremental atrial and ventricular pacing and extrastimulus testing from the right atrium and right ventricle are performed to further delineate the electrophysiological properties of the AP and induction of reentrant tachycardia. If sustained tachycardia cannot be induced, isoprenalin can be infused to facilitate tachycardia induction.

Cryoablation catheters

Deflectable, 7 French-sized cryoablation catheters with a 4 mm tip (Freezor, Medtronic, MN, USA) or 6 mm tip (Freezor Xtra, Medtronic, MN, USA) are commonly used for the treatment of APs. Cryomapping function is available for these catheters. In our center, we had the experience of using a 9 French-sized deflectable 8 mm tip cryoablation catheter (Freezor Max, Medtronic, MN, USA) in the treatment of LFW APs. Although this catheter delivers higher freezing power, a cryomapping function is not available. The cryoablation catheter is composed of an outer shaft maintained under constant vacuum and an inner injection tube through which

liquid N$_2$O is injected. The liquid N$_2$O escapes from the end of the injection tube at the tip of the catheter shaft into the outer lumen and evaporates, resulting in cooling of the tip by the Joule–Thompson effect. Gaseous N$_2$O is then vented from the outer shaft to a reservoir outside the body. A thermocouple at the catheter tip enables monitoring of its temperature.

Cryomapping and cryoablation protocol for APs

Similar to RFCA, the target site for cryoablation can be located by the identification of an isolated AP potential[40] or presence of other electrogram criteria.[5] At the target ablation site, the temperature of the tip of the cryoablation catheter can be lowered to −30 °C to perform cryomapping. Cryomapping is successful if there is no inadvertent AVB, plus one of the following: (1) the disappearance of the delta wave on a surface electrocardiogram (ECG) for APs with anterograde conduction (Figure 8.1), or (2) a change from an eccentric to concentric pattern of conduction during ventricular pacing for APs with only retrograde conduction (Figure 8.2). Cryomapping should be maintained for 60 s to look for occurrence of inadvertent AVB. The time-to-effect of cryomapping or cryoablation is preferably within 20 s. With successful cryomapping, cryoablation can be started by lowering the temperature of the catheter tip to −75 °C. The duration of an application of cryoablation is 4 min. A freeze–thaw cycle (i.e., another 4 min cryoablation repeated at the same site after rewarming from the first 4 min of cryoapplication) can be given to increase the size and permanency of the lesion.

Performance of catheter cryoablation of APs

Efficacy, safety, and recurrence in general

The data on the performance of catheter cryoablation in treating APs are scarce. Studies with small numbers of patients have been performed in both adult and pediatric populations (Table 8.2).[41–44] In some of these studies, recurrence rates have not been reported in detail. However, cryocatheters with tip sizes ranging from 4 to 8 mm have been used in different studies. In general, a lower acute procedural success rate compared to that of RFCA was reported. The acute procedural success rates varied from 60% to 87%. In particular, in the largest

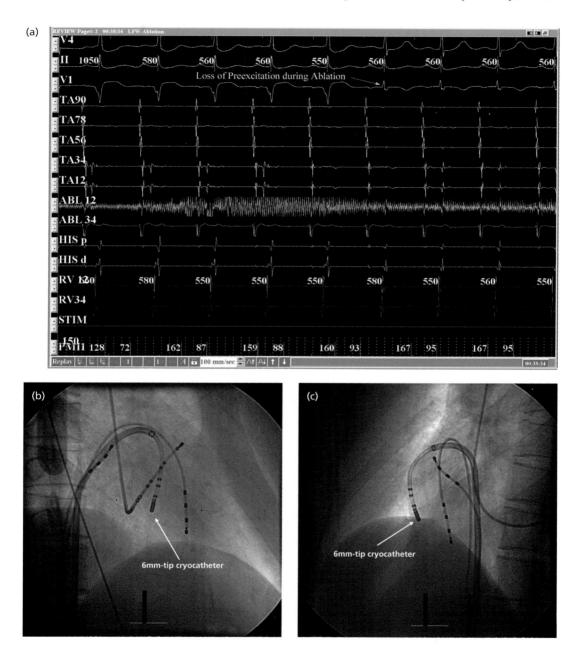

Figure 8.1. Catheter cryoablation of a right free wall accessory pathway with a 6 mm tip catheter. (a) Loss of preexcitation during ablation. Note the classical artifacts in the ablation channel due to ice ball formation at the catheter tip. (b) Fluoroscopic position of the ablation catheter in the right anterior oblique (RAO) view. (c) Fluoroscopic position of the ablation catheter in the left anterior oblique (LAO) view.

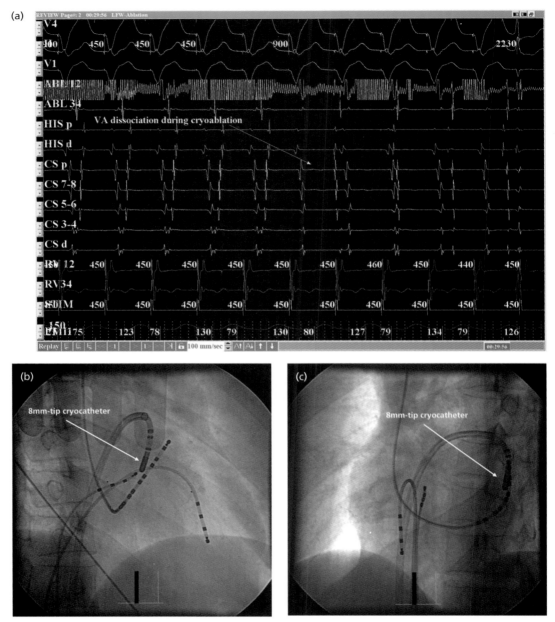

Figure 8.2. Catheter cryoablation of a left free wall accessory pathway with an 8 mm tip catheter via the transseptal approach. (a) Retrograde conduction pattern converted from eccentricity to ventriculo-atrial dissociation. Note the classical artifacts in the ablation channel due to ice ball formation at the catheter tip. (b) Fluoroscopic position of the ablation catheter in the right anterior oblique (RAO) view. (c) Fluoroscopic position of the ablation catheter in the left anterior oblique (LAO) view.

Table 8.2. Performance of catheter cryoablation in the treatment of accessory pathways

Authors	Acute procedural success				Permanent atrioventricular block				Recurrence			
	All (%)	LFW (%)	RFW (%)	Septal (%)	All (%)	LFW (%)	RFW (%)	Septal (%)	All (%)	LFW (%)	RFW (%)	Septal (%)
Friedman (2004)[42] (n = 50; 4 mm#)	38 (76)	15 (65)	2 (100)	21 (84)	0	0	0	0	N/A	N/A	N/A	N/A
Chan (2007)[43] (n = 23; 6 or 8 mm#)	20 (87)	15 (88)	5 (83)	N/A	0	0	0	0	1 (5)	1 (7)	0	N/A
Kirsh* (2005)[44] (n = 30; 4 or 6 mm#)	18 (60)	6 (43)##		12 (75)	0	0	0	0	N/A	N/A	N/A	N/A
Kriebel* (2005)[45] (n = 23; 4 or 6 mm#)	15 (65)	8 (80)	4 (57)	3 (50)	0	0	0	0	2 (13)	0	1 (25)	1 (33)

LFW: left free wall; N: number of accessory pathways; N/A: not available or not applicable; RFW: right free wall. #refers to size of cryocatheter; ##refers to combined data on LFW and RFW accessory pathways.
*Study performed in paediatric patients;

series reported by Friedman *et al.*, a very low acute procedural success rate of only 65% was achieved by using a 4 mm tip cryocatheter to treat left free wall APs.[41] The exact reason for this observation is still unclear. A possible explanation may be that cryoablation produces a smaller lesion[34] due to its biophysical properties and the phenomenon of cryoadhesion. The lesion size in the left heart, compared to the right heart, may be further reduced because of higher blood flow in the former. Chan *et al.* achieved a relatively higher acute procedural success rate of 88% for LFW AP ablation by using an 8 mm tip cryocatheter, which produces a larger lesion.[42]

No permanent inadvertent AVB occurred in the treatment of septal APs by cryoablation. The limited data on the recurrence rate preclude any meaningful conclusion in this aspect. However, according to my experience, the recurrence rate is comparable to that of RFCA for RFW and septal APs. In contrast, for LFW APs, the recurrence rate is still significantly higher than that of RFCA, even with the use of an 8 mm tip cryocatheter.

A closer look at catheter cryoablation of septal APs

The primary advantage of catheter cryoablation is the ability to create a more focused lesion and the availability of the cryomapping function. These properties make it the energy of choice in the ablation of septal APs (Figure 8.3). Gaita *et al.* reported their experience of catheter cryoablation in 11 paraHisian and 9 midseptal APs.[45] An acute procedural success rate of 100% was achieved. Four (20%) patients had recurrence of AP conduction, and they were all successfully reablated with cryothermic energy. Most important of all, there was no complication of inadvertent permanent AVB. Atienza *et al.* reported their experience in catheter cryoablation in 22 patients with midseptal or paraHisian APs.[46] Twelve patients had midseptal APs, and 10 patients had paraHisian APs. Eight of the patients underwent RFCA unsuccessfully. Cryoablation was successfully performed in 20 patients, with an acute procedural success rate of 91%. No permanent AVB was observed, and there were two patients with permanent right bundle branch block after cryoablation. Three (15%) patients had recurrence of AP conduction, and two of them underwent repeat cryoablation successfully.

Catheter cryoablation of epicardial APs through the coronary sinus

Left-sided AP may uncommonly be located epicardially. In a study involving 212 patients with left free wall APs, multiple endocardial RFCA failed in 8 (4%) of them.[47] The investigators attempted RFCA inside the coronary sinus (CS) and achieved acute procedural success in seven (88%) of those patients. However, all patients experienced marked pain during ablation. In six patients, the ablation catheter remained adherent to the CS wall despite significant mechanical traction, and new energy delivery was required for retrieval of the catheter to decrease the risk of venous rupture. In two patients, CS thrombus was observed after ablation. Giorgberidze *et al.* has also reported RFCA inside the CS in 12 patients with 14 APs located in the left posteroseptal or free wall region.[48] The acute procedural success rate was 71%, and there was no recurrence or complication. In an animal study performed by Langberg *et al.*, RF energy applied inside the CS resulted in CS thrombosis in three dogs but no collateral damage to the left circumflex artery.[49] In contrast, Huang *et al.* found damage to the branches of the underlying coronary artery with necrotizing arteritis and arterial sclerosis in 2 out of 20 dogs receiving RFCA inside the CS.[50] Although still controversial, RFCA inside the CS should be regarded as involving extra risks.

Catheter cryoablation may be a safer approach for ablation inside the CS (Figure 8.4). Collins *et al.* described 21 pediatric patients with left-sided APs and cryoablation inside the CS.[51] They achieved an acute procedural success rate of 71%. The recurrence rate was 40%. Most importantly, there was no evidence of coronary artery damage after the procedure.

Cryomapping failure

Cryomapping is a unique property of cryoablation. However, it is clear from the biophysical property of the energy source that the ultimate effect of cryoablation may not be totally predicted by cryomapping. Khairy *et al.* has shown that the lower the temperature, the deeper the cryolesion will be.[33] With each 10 °C decrease in the nadir temperature, the depth of a cryolesion can be increased by 0.4 mm. Skanes *et al.* reported that in 4 out of 12 patients with AVNRT, cryomapping at a temperature of −28 °C failed to produce conduction block in the slow

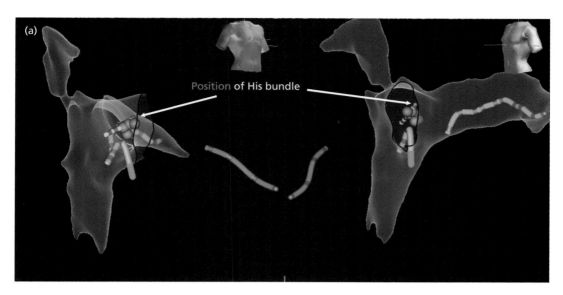

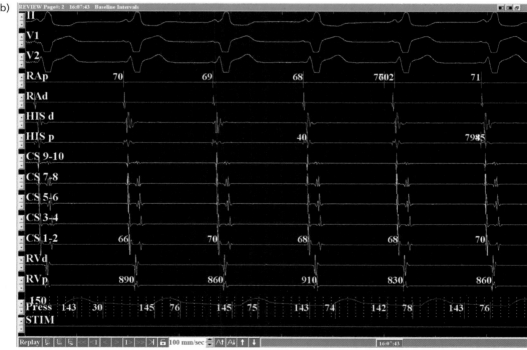

Figure 8.3. Catheter cryoablation with a 6 mm tip catheter in a patient with multiple right-sided accessory pathways, including a paraHisian pathway. (a) Catheter positions recorded from the Ensite Velocity system (St. Jude Medical, MN, USA). Views are shown in right anterior oblique (RAO) (left) and left anterior oblique (LAO) (right) projections. Diagnostic electrode catheters are shown in blue (coronary sinus), yellow (His bundle), and red (right ventricular apex), respectively. The 6 mm tip cryocatheter is shown in orange. Round dots of different colors represent cryolesions. (b) Baseline intracardiac electrograms during sinus rhythm with fused atrial and ventricular electrograms at the His channel. (c) Intracardiac electrograms during sinus rhythm after cryoablation at the paraHisian region. The separation of the atrial and ventricular electrograms in the His channel indicates conduction block in the paraHisian accessory pathway. There is a change in the pre-excitation pattern on surface electrocardiograms (ECG). The persistence of pre-excitation despite successful cryoablation of the paraHisian accessory pathway indicates the presence of other pathway(s).

(c)

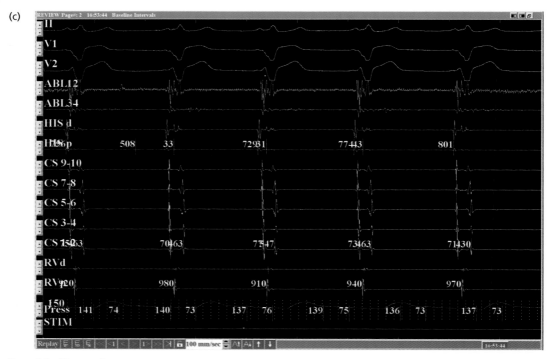

Figure 8.3. (*Continued*)

pathway.[52] However, by lowering the temperature to −37 to −52 °C at the same site, the slow pathway could be blocked. On the other hand, Fischbach *et al.* observed that in 5 out of 32 patients with different kinds of supraventricular arrhythmias, reversible AVB still occurred with cryoablation despite its absence during cryomapping.[53] In a case series, three out of nine patients with septal APs had cryomapping failure.[54] Two patients had successful cryoablation at sites with ineffective cryomapping, while one patient experienced reversible AVB with cryoablation despite its absence during cryomapping. All these observations highlight the importance of avoiding complete reliance on the function of cryomapping. With optimal conventional mapping criteria, cryoablation may be successful despite ineffective cryomapping. Likewise, one has to remain vigilant for AVB during cryoablation even if it has not occurred during cryomapping.

Conclusions

Radiofrequency has been the gold standard energy source for catheter ablation of APs with, in general,

high acute procedural success, low complication, and low recurrence rates. However, lower acute procedural success and higher recurrence rates have been observed in RFCA of septal APs. Most importantly, there is a substantial risk of inadvertent AVB. Uncommon complications of collateral damage to coronary arteries and autonomic nerves are also of concern. Cryothermy is an alternative source of energy that is characterized by a more discrete and accurate lesion with preservation of the endothelial layer. The unique properties of cryomapping and cryoadhesion further improve the safety profile of this energy source. Currently, the data on the performance of cryoablation for the treatment of APs are relatively scarce. In general, a lower acute procedural success rate has been observed, especially for left-sided APs. Recurrence rates may be similar for both energy sources for RFW and septal APs, but it remains higher in cryoablation for LFW APs. Cryoablation is especially preferred in the treatment of septal APs because of an extremely low, if not zero, risk of inadvertent AVB. Lastly, cryoablation may also be considered in treating left-sided epicardial APs when ablation inside the CS is required.

(a)

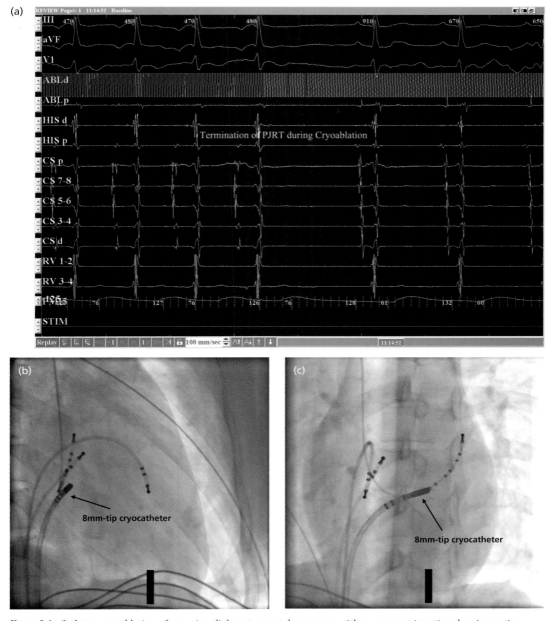

Figure 8.4. Catheter cryoablation of an epicardial posteroseptal accessory with permanent junctional reciprocating tachycardia (PJRT) with an 8 mm tip catheter. (a) Termination of PJRT during cryoablation at the ostium of the coronary sinus. Note the classical artifacts in the ablation channel due to ice ball formation at the catheter tip. (b) Fluoroscopic position of the ablation catheter in the right anterior oblique (RAO) view. (c) Fluoroscopic position of the ablation catheter in the left anterior oblique (LAO) view.

Interactive Case Studies related to this chapter can be found at this book's companion website, at **www.chancryoablation.com**

References

1. Blomström-Lundqvist C, Scheinman MM, Aliot EM, *et al.* ACC/AHA/ESC guidelines for the management of patients with supraventricular arrhythmias. J Am Coll Cardiol. 2003;42:1493–31.

2. Jackman WM, Wang XZ, Friday KJ, *et al.* Catheter ablation of accessory pathways (Wolff–Parkinson–White syndrome) by radiofrequency current. N Engl J Med. 1991;334:1605–11.

3. Kuck KH, Schlüter M, Geiger M, *et al.* Radiofrequency current catheter ablation of accessory atrioventricular pathways. Lancet. 1991;337:1557–61.

4. Calkins H, Sousa J, el Atassi R, *et al.* Diagnosis and cure of the Wolff–Parkinson–White syndrome or paroxysmal supraventricular tachycardia during a single electrophysiologic test. N Engl J Med. 1991;324:1612–18.

5. Lesh MD, van Hare GF, Schamp DJ, *et al.* Curative percutaneous catheter ablation using radiofrequency energy for accessory pathways in all locations: results in 100 consecutive patients. J Am Coll Cardiol. 1992;19:1303–9.

6. Kay GN, Epstein AE, Dailey SM, *et al.* Role of radiofrequency ablation in the management of supraventricular arrhythmias: experience in 760 consecutive patients. J Cardiovasc Electrophysiol. 1993;4:371–89.

7. Swartz JF, Tracy CM, Fletcher RD, *et al.* Radiofrequency endocardial catheter ablation of accessory atrioventricular pathway atrial insertion sites. Circulation. 1993;87:487–99.

8. Hindricks G. The Multicentre European Radiofrequency Survey (MERFS): complications of radiofrequency catheter ablation of arrhythmias. Eur Heart J. 1993;14:1644–53.

9. Scheinman MM. NASPE survey on catheter ablation. Pacing Clin Electrophysiol. 1995;18:1474–8.

10. Calkins H, Yong P, Miller JM, *et al.* Catheter ablation of accessory pathways, atrioventricular nodal reentrant tachycardia and the atrioventricular junction: final results of a prospective, multicenter clinical trial. Circulation. 1999;99:262–70.

11. Dagres N, Clague JR, Breithardt G, *et al.* Significant gender differences in radiofrequency catheter ablation therapy. J Am Coll Cardiol. 2003;42:1103–7.

12. Kobza R, Kottkamp H, Piorkowski C, *et al.* Radiofrequency ablation of accessory pathways: contempo-rary success rates and complications in 323 patients. Zeit Kardiol. 2005;94:193–9.

13. Schneider HE, Kriebel T, Gravenhorst VD, *et al.* Incidence of coronary artery injury immediately after catheter ablation for supraventricular tachycardias in infants and children. Heart Rhythm. 2009;6:461–7.

14. Spar DS, Silver ES, Hordof AJ, *et al.* Coronary artery spasm during radiofrequency ablation of a left lateral accessory pathway. Pediatr Cardiol. 2010;31: 724–7.

15. Khanal S, Ribeiro PA, Platt M, *et al.* Right coronary artery occlusion as a complication of accessory pathway ablation in a 12-year-old treated with stenting. Catheter Cardiovasc Interv. 1999;46:59–61.

16. Hosaka Y, Chinushi M, Takahashi K, *et al.* Coronary vasospasm triggered ventricular fibrillation delayed after radiofrequency ablation of the right accessory pathway. Europace. 2009;11:1554–6.

17. Dinckal H, Yucel O, Kirilmaz A, *et al.* Left anterior descending coronary artery occlusion after left lateral free wall accessory pathway ablation: what is the possible mechanism? Europace. 2003;5:263–6.

18. Moreira JM, Curimbaba J, Filho HC, *et al.* Persistent inappropriate sinus tachycardia after radiofrequency ablation of left lateral accessory pathway. J Cardiovasc Electrophysiol. 2006;17:678–81.

19. Jinbo Y, Kobayashi Y, Miyata A, *et al.* Decreasing parasympathetic tone activity and proarrhythmic effect after radiofrequency catheter ablation-differences in ablation site. Jpn Circ J. 1998;62:733–40.

20. Emkanjoo Z, Alasti M, Arya A, *et al.* Heart rate variability: does it change after RF ablation of reentrant supraventricular tachycardia? J Interv Cardiac Electrophysiol. 2005;14:147–51.

21. Psychari SN, Theodorakis GN, Koutelou M, *et al.* Cardiac denervation after radiofrequency ablation of supraventricular tachycardias. Am J Cardiol. 1998; 81:725–31.

22. Shiraishi H, Shirayama T, Yoshida S, *et al.* Transient complete atrioventricular block during catheter ablation of left free wall bypass tract. Jpn Circ J. 2000; 64:399–403.

23. Ehlert FA, Goldberger JJ, Brooks R, *et al.* Persistent inappropriate sinus tachycardia after radiofrequency current catheter modification of the atrioventricular node. Am J Cardiol. 1992;69:1092–5.

24. Frey B, Heinz G, Kreiner G, *et al.* Increased heart rate variability after radiofrequency ablation. Am J Cardiol. 1993;71:1460–1.

25. Chen SA, Chiang CE, Tai CT, *et al.* Complications of diagnostic electrophysiological studies and radiofrequency catheter ablation in patients with tachyarrhythmias: an eight year survey of 3966 consecutive

procedures in a tertiary referral center. Am J Cardiol. 1996;77:41–6.

26. Kocovic DZ, Harada T, Shea J, et al. Alterations of heart rate and heart rate variability after radiofrequency catheter ablation of supraventricular tachycardia. Delineation of parasympathetic pathways in the human heart. Circulation. 1993;88(Pt. 1): 1671–81.

27. Chiang CE, Chen SA, Wang DC, et al. Arrhythmogenicity of catheter ablation in supraventricular tachycardia. Am Heart J. 1993;125:388–95.

28. Psychari SN, et al. Cardiac denervation after radiofrequency ablation of supraventricular tachycardias. Am J Cardiol. 1998;81:725–31.

29. Jinbo Y, Kobayashi Y, Miyata A, et al. Decreasing parasympathetic tone activity and proarrhythmic effect after radiofrequency catheter ablation. Differences in ablations site. Jpn Circ J. 1998;62:733–40.

30. Stamato NJ, Eddy SL, Whiting DJ. Transient complete heart block during radiofrequency ablation of a left lateral bypass tract. Pacing Clin Electrophysiol. 1996; 19:1351–4.

31. Singh B, Sudan D, Kaul U. Transient atrioventricular block following radiofrequency ablation of left free wall accessory pathway. J Interv Cardiac Electrophysiol. 1998;2:305–7.

32. Shiraishi H, Shirayama T, Yoshida S, et al. Transient complete atrioventricular block during catheter ablation of left free wall bypass tract. Jpn Circ J. 2000; 64:399–403.

33. Khairy P, Dubuc M. Transcatheter cryoablation part I: preclinical experience. Pacing Clin Electrophysiol. 2008;31:112–20.

34. Khairy P, Chauvet P, Lehmann J, et al. Lower incidence of thrombus formation with cryoenergy versus radiofrequency catheter ablation. Circulation. 2003; 107:2045–50.

35. Aoyama H, Nakagawa H, Pitha JV, et al. Comparison of cryothermia and radiofrequency current in safety and efficacy of catheter ablation within the canine coronary sinus close to the left circumflex coronary artery. J Cardiovasc Electrophysiol. 2005; 16:1218–26.

36. Skanes AC, Jones DL, Teefy P, et al. Safety and feasibility of cryothermal ablation within the mid and distal coronary sinus. J Cardiovasc Electrophysiol. 2004;15: 1319–23.

37. Rodriguez LM, Leunissen J, Hoekstra A, et al. Transvenous cold mapping and cryoablation of the AV node in dogs: observations of chronic lesions and comparison to those obtained with radiofrequency ablation. J Cardiovasc Electrophysiol. 1998;9: 1055–61.

38. Dubuc M, Roy D, Thibault B, et al. Transvenous catheter ice mapping and cryoablation of the atrioventricular node in dogs. Pacing Clin Electrophysiol. 1999;22:1488–98.

39. Dubuc M, Talajic M, Roy D, et al. Feasibility of cardiac cryoablation using a transvenous steerable electrical catheter. J Interv Cardiac Electrophysiol. 1998;2: 285–92.

40. Nakagawa H, Jackman WM. Catheter ablation of paroxysmal supraventricular tachycardia. Circulation. 2007;116:2465–78.

41. Friedman PL, Dubuc M, Green MS, et al. Catheter cryoablation of supraventricular tachycardia: results of the multicenter prospective "frosty" trial. Heart Rhythm. 2004;1:129–38.

42. Chan NY, Lau CL, Lo YK, et al. Catheter cryoablation as the primary treatment for cardiac arrhythmias. Chin J Cardiac Pacing Electrophysiol. 2007;21: 132–6.

43. Kirsch JA, Gross GJ, O'Connor S, et al. Transcatheter cryoablation of tachyarrhythmias in children. J Am Coll Cardiol. 2005;45:133–6.

44. Kriebel T, Broistedt C, Kroll M, et al. Efficacy and safety of cryoenergy in the ablation of atrioventricular reentrant tachycardia substrate in children and adolescents. J Cardiovasc Electrophysiol. 2005;16: 960–6.

45. Gaita F, Riccardi R, Hocini M, et al. Safety and efficacy of cryoablation of accessory pathways adjacent to the normal conduction system. J Cardiovasc Electrophysiol. 2003;14:825–9.

46. Atienza F, Arenal A, Torrecilla EG, et al. Acute and long term outcome of transvenous cryoablation of midseptal and paraHisian accessory pathways in patients at high risk of atrioventricular block during radiofrequency ablation. Amer J Cardiol. 2004;93: 1302–5.

47. Haissaguerre M, Gaita F, Fischer B, et al. Radiofrequency catheter ablation of left lateral accessory pathways via the coronary sinus. Circulation. 1992; 86:1464–8.

48. Giorgberidze I, Saksena S, Krol RB, et al. Efficacy and safety of radiofrequency catheter ablation of left-sided accessory pathways through the coronary sinus. Am J Cardiol. 1995;76:359–65.

49. Langbery J, Griffin JC, Herre JM, et al. Catheter ablation of accessory pathways using radiofrequency energy in the canine coronary sinus. J Am Coll Cardiol. 1989;13:491–6.

50. Huang SK, Graham AR, Bharati S, et al. Short and long-term effects of transcatheter ablation of the coronary sinus by radiofrequency energy. Circulation. 1988;78:416–27.

51. Collins KK, Rhee EK, Kirsh JA, *et al.* Cryoablation of accessory pathways in the coronary sinus in young patients: a multicenter study from the Pediatric and Congenital Electrophysiology Society's Working Group on cryoablation. J Cardiovasc Electrophysiol. 2007;18:592–7.

52. Skanes AC, Dubuc M, Klein GJ, *et al.* Cryothermal ablation of the slow pathway for the elimination of atrioventricular nodal reentrant tachycardia. Circulation. 2000;102:2856–60.

53. Fischbach PS, Saarel E, Dick M 2nd. Transient atrioventricular conduction block with cryoablation following normal cryomapping. Heart Rhythm. 2004;1:554–7.

54. Reddy VK, Villuendas R, Rudin A, *et al.* Cryomap failure. J Interv Cardiac Electrophysiol. 2007;19:139–41.

CHAPTER 9

Catheter Cryoablation for the Treatment of Ventricular Arrhythmias

Luigi Di Biase,[1,2,3,4] Xue Yan,[1,2] Pasquale Santangeli,[1,3,5] Amin Al-Ahmad,[5] Henry H. Hsia,[5] David J. Burkhardt,[1] and Andrea Natale[1,2,5,6]

[1]Texas Cardiac Arrhythmia Institute at St. David's Medical Center, Austin, TX, USA
[2]University of Texas, Austin, TX, USA
[3]University of Foggia, Foggia, Italy
[4]Albert Einstein College of Medicine at Montefiore Hospital, New York, NY, USA
[5]Stanford University School of Medicine, Palo Alto, CA, USA
[6]Sutter Pacific Medical Center, San Francisco, CA, USA

Introduction

Catheter ablation is a viable therapeutic option for the treatment of ventricular arrhythmia (VA) in patients with either a "normal" heart or cardiomyopathy.[1–3]

A number of ablation energy modalities have been used in an effort to eliminate arrhythmias, including unipolar radiofrequency (RF) energy, irrigated and non-irrigated bipolar RF energy, microwave, laser, cryoenergy, and ultrasound ablation.

RF energy is currently the most utilized energy source for the treatment of VAs, especially in the settings of scar-related ventricular tachycardia (VT).[1–3] Although advancements in the technology and the understanding of the pathophysiology have allowed electrophysiologists to accomplish even more in the treatment of VAs using RF energy, there are still many limitations to the use of this technique, which motivates research into alternative sources of ablation energy.[4]

Cryoenergy has been used during surgical procedures for decades in different ways. Differently from RF catheter ablation (RFCA), in which heat destroys cells by coagulation and tissue necrosis with potential thrombus formation and aneurysmal dilatation, cryoablation involves a distinct pathophysiological process.[5] As such, it carries a unique safety and efficacy profile and provides an interesting alternative to RFCA in certain instances. While appealing, the use of cryoenergy as the primary energy source for the treatment of VAs has not been widely established or reported. By searching the literature, only a few case studies and two large series aimed to evaluate the feasibility and safety of cryoablation for the treatment of VAs can be found.[6–8]

This chapter will examine the use of cryoenergy as an alternative source for the treatment of VAs.

History of cryoablation

Although the application of cryoenergy for surgical purposes has been employed for several decades, harnessing this energy into a steerable transcatheter format represents a relatively recent landmark in arrhythmia therapy.

Cooling cryosurgical devices were first introduced in the early 1960s.[9] This introduction was rapidly followed by several pertinent advancements. In 1964, Lister *et al.* first described the application

The Practice of Catheter Cryoablation for Cardiac Arrhythmias, First Edition. Edited by Ngai-Yin Chan.
© 2014 John Wiley & Sons, Ltd. Published 2014 by John Wiley & Sons, Ltd.

of cryoenergy to the cardiac conduction tissue by suturing a 4 mm U-shaped silver tube near the bundle of His.[10] Next, in 1977, Harrison et al. performed the first cardiac cryosurgery with handheld bipolar electrode probes.[11] He conducted his study initially in 20 dogs with atrioventricular (AV) nodal ablation, then in three patients with refractory supraventricular tachycardia. Complete but reversible AV block was achieved in all patients with the application of the probe at the His bundle site at 0 °C. Permanent, complete AV block was achieved when the applied probe temperature was further lowered to −60 °C. In 1984, Klein et al. followed with a larger series study with longer-term follow-up.[12] A refrigerated −60 °C handheld cryoprobe was applied at the site where intraoperative mapping localized the arrhythmogenic substrate. The effectiveness was evaluated during continuous monitoring of the cardiac electrical activity. AV block was successfully achieved in 17 of 22 patients. Significant engineering advances in the 1990s allowed for the development of systems for cryoablation that shared similarities with the standard ablation catheters for RF energy delivery. This system consisted of a steerable catheter and a cryoablation console. With these advancements, in 2001, Dubuc et al. was able to conduct the first clinical study with transcatheter cryoablation.[13]

Cryoablation technology

The goal of cryoablation is to destroy targeted cells by freezing the tissue in a discrete and focused manner. Ablation using cryoenergy relies on the Joule–Thompson effect. At high pressure, a refrigerant such as nitrous oxide (N_2O) flows down a hollow injection tube to the tip of the catheter (or probe). The pressure is lower in the tip's outer shaft, so the liquid refrigerant will expand to a gas, causing the tip to cool. As cryoenergy is delivered and heat is extracted from the electrode–tissue interface, the catheter tip will eventually adhere tightly to the surrounding tissue (known as the cryoadherence effect). Gas is constantly removed from a second, vacuumed tube inside the catheter. Due to the need for both a pump and a vacuum system, cryo systems are typically contained in relatively large consoles. N_2O is provided under pressure through encased cylinders. While heat is extracted from the tissue interface, the console constantly monitors the fluid

flow in the catheter. By adjusting the flow rate of the refrigerant, the tip temperature can be precisely controlled.

Two cryoablation systems are currently available.[4] One is by Cryocath Technologies Inc. (QB, Canada), and the second is by CryoCor Inc. (CA, USA). The Cryocath system has steerable catheters that are 7 or 9 French size with a 4, 6, or 8 mm long tip electrode. The console for this system has an algorithm for cryomapping (slow decrease of temperature to −30 °C for up to 80 s) and an algorithm for cryoablation (faster decrease of temperature to −75 °C for up to 480 s). The target temperature can also be manually preset on the console within the range of −30 to −75 °C. The other cryoablation system by CryoCor has steerable catheters that are 10 French size with 6.5 or 10 mm long tip electrodes. Its console has a built-in closed-loop precooler for the nitrous oxide. The flow rate is adjusted during application to maintain a temperature of −80 °C.[4]

Lesion formation by cryothermal energy

Before widespread application of cryosurgical devices, Hass and Taylor et al. wrote initial descriptions of controlled myocardial lesions made with cryoenergy using carbon dioxide as the refrigerant.[14] Lesions were notably described as homogeneous and sharply demarcated with preserved structural integrity. These initial descriptions of tissue characteristics remain valid today.

The mechanisms underlying cryoenergy lesion formation occur through both direct cell injury and vascular-mediated tissue injury. Depending on the temperature range that the cells are cooled to, various degrees of direct cellular injury can be achieved. At mild temperatures (0 to −20 °C), ice will only form extracellularly.[9]

Extracellular ice formation makes the environment hyperosmotic and causes water to shift from the intracellular to extracellular. This shift generates cellular shrinkage and damage to the membrane. If the application is prolonged, cooling within this temperature range may result in cellular death. However, short ablation applications within this range are generally reversible with minimal cellular damage. Clinically this ability is used as cryomapping. With further cooling (temperatures down to −40 to −70 °C), cryoablation will result in intracellular ice formation. The formation of intracellular ice leads to irreversible organelle and cell membrane disruption, as well as cell death.[15] In addition to direct cellular injury, as the tissue is frozen by cryoablation, circulation in the tissue will decrease and cease uniformly in the frozen tissue. Although tissue damage due to this is indistinguishable from that due to intracellular ice formation, vasoconstriction can also potentially lead to cell death. Upon rewarming of the tissue after cryoenergy application, regional hyperthermia ensues, with increased vascular permeability and edema formation.[9]

Cryoenergy versus RF energy: clinical implications

RFCA can be used to create larger and deeper lesions than cryoablation. The lesions that cryoablation creates are smaller and more localized, which is often insufficient for ensuring long-term ablation success.[6]

Cryoablation requires longer ablation times to eliminate potentials, and the procedure also has a higher rate of recurrence. In addition, due to the specific aspects required of cryoenergy delivery, the cryocatheter is also stiffer. This results in hindered maneuverability and limits the use of the cryocatheter in areas such as the coronary sinus branches. Despite the fact that many of these aspects are the shortcomings of the use of cryothermal ablation, these characteristic limitations also contribute to the factors that make cryoablation advantageous in certain cases.

There are many difficulties associated with using RFCA. With RFCA, it is difficult to test the ablation target while applying energy and there are issues with catheter stability. In addition, using the RF ablation catheter for long durations of time and attempting to create continuous linear lesions may result in local thrombosis or ulcerative lesions. Another problem is that the effect of RF application cannot be predicted until after a permanent lesion has been created. This has important implications for ablation procedures involving tissues close to areas such as the AV node, where permanent AV block is a potential complication. Alternatively, the use of cryoablation produces delineated, homogeneous lesions with the absence of ulcerations, thrombus formation, and even inflammation. Creating cryolesions preserves the underlying tissue architecture and results in minimal endothelial and endocardial disruption and a low risk of perfora-

tion. Part of this is likely due to the cryoadherence effect of cryoablation. There is not a similar parallel for cryoadherence while using RFCA. While using RFCA, the catheter tip does not adhere to the tissue. This often results in inconsistent linear lesions and necessitates multiple applications. This is a major shortcoming of RFCA. Overall, it is important to maintain fixed and stable contact during ablation applications, especially in proximity to critical areas such as the AV node and His bundle. During cryoablation, since the catheter is tightly adhered to the targeted tissue, the lesion produced is very localized, and there is no additional "brushing" of the tip electrode (commonly observed during RFCA).

Although it is faster to produce lesions with RFCA, its irreversible effects also make the process rather unforgiving. The longer ablation duration required by the use of cryoablation may be more clinically useful for modulating lesion formation in critical areas such as near the AV node or His bundle.[9] Unlike with RFCA, if inadvertent modifications of conduction over normal pathways are observed during cryoablation application, cessation of ablation results in a return to baseline conduction properties with low likelihood of permanent damage to the normal conduction. While the reversibility of cryoablation is adverse to the ultimate goals of the arrhythmia treatment, its effects are very useful during the ablation procedures.[4]

Cryoablation in the settings of VT ablation: clinical studies

Only a few case studies and two large series aimed to evaluate the feasibility and safety of cryoablation for the treatment of VAs.

In 2010, Timmermans et al.[7] reported on the feasibility and safety of cryoablation for the treatment of postinfarction and idiopathic VTs. The report included VA ablation in 17 patients (15 men and 2 women, 58+/−18 years): 10 patients had postinfarction VT, while the remaining 7 had idiopathic VT. The study had only a short-term follow-up of 6 months. No complication was reported, and the success rate was 60% in the postinfarction VT group and 86% in the idiopathic VT group. Switch to manual ablation was required in two patients for the presence of hemodynamically unstable VT. This study demonstrated the feasibility of catheter-based cryoablation for the treatment of postinfarction VT. This study also used a slightly larger test group to replicate the results of previous cases of cryoablation of idiopathic VT.[16]

Rather than focus on the applicability of cryothermy to various structures, this study examined the effectiveness and safety of cryoablation for the treatment of monomorphic, right- or left-sided, postinfarction, and idiopathic VT. A previous study has already shown its effectiveness in right-sided VT. Since the only complication that resulted from this study was unrelated to the cryocatheter, this study confirmed the safety of using cryoablation. The study concluded that cryoablation was also an effective method of treatment for VAs, since the overall acute efficacy was 100%. Although there was a short period of follow-up after the procedure, the insight that this study gave on the long-term efficacy is limited.

In 2011, Di Biase et al.[6] reported on 33 cases where cryoablation of VAs was attempted as the initial strategy or was considered to prevent potential damage to other structures such as the coronary arteries, the phrenic nerve, and the His bundle. Of the 33 patients (54% male and 46% female, 54+/−8 years) included in the study, 25 patients had normal hearts with preserved ejection fraction, while the other 8 had ischemic and nonischemic

cardiomyopathy. At the long-term follow-up (24 months), all 15 patients with acute procedural success by cryoablation were free from recurrence of clinical VAs. Eight (out of nine) patients who failed cryoablation as the primary energy source underwent a second procedure with RF.

As shown in the studies discussed here, although it has some technical limitations cryoablation proved to be advantageous. Importantly, along with creating smaller lesions, cryoablation makes sharp, delineated homogeneous lesions and produces less endothelial disruption, which will better preserve the extracellular collagen and minimize thrombus formation, inflammation, and pain to the patient in comparison to RFCA.

Cryoablation has the important advantage of reducing the risk of damage to surrounding structures during ablation application, such as when it is in close proximity to the conduction system, phrenic nerve, and coronary arteries. These are important factors to consider when ablating near the His bundle and other vessels that are encased by only a thin layer of connective tissue. This trait was explored largely in our study.[6]

In the case of paraHisian VT ablation (Figures 9.1 and 9.2), the study results suggest that cryoab-

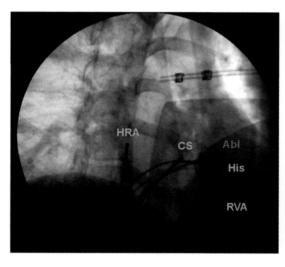
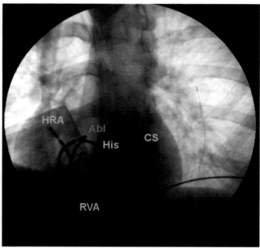

RAO   LAO

Figure 9.1. Fluoroscopy of the same patients described in Figure 9.2 showing the catheter positions. Left: right anterior oblique (RAO) view; right: left anterior oblique (LAO) view. The distance between the ablation catheter and the His region is 3.3 mm. HRA: high right atrium catheter; CS: coronary sinus catheter; His: His bundle catheter; RVA: right ventricular apex catheter; Abl: ablation catheter. Note the close proximity of the ablation and His bundle catheters (paraHisian).

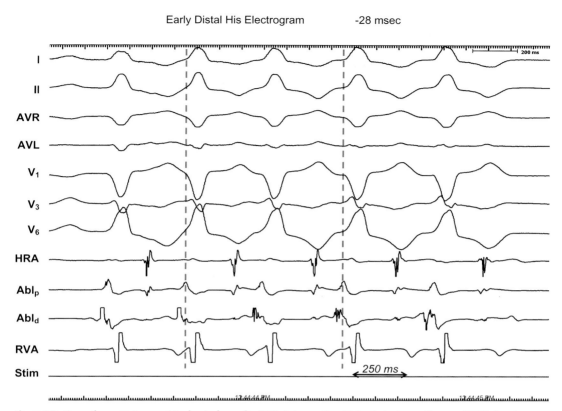

Figure 9.2. Case of paraHisian ventricular tachycardia (VT). Intracardiac 12-lead electrocardiogram (ECG) showing nonsustained VT with left bundle branch block (LBBB)-like QRS with tall, smoothly contoured R-waves in the inferior ECG leads. The local ventricular activation at the distal His region (abld) is −28 ms earlier than the QRS initiation on the ECG. From top to bottom: surface ECG leads I, II, AVR, AVL, V1, V3, and V6; electrogram recorded from ablation proximal (Ablp) and distal (Abld) at the level of the His, right ventricular apex (RVA).

lation should be considered as an optional first-line approach. In reference to ablation of the aortic cusps, RF ablations at sites close to the AV node have not been attempted or have resulted in complete AV block, so the study results suggest that cryoablation of the aortic cusps should be considered the first-line approach, at least in younger patients. Importantly, caution should be taken to avoid dissection in the aortic root due to the stiffness of the cryocatheter (Figure 9.3).

Premature ventricular contractions (PVCs) and VTs may arise from the interventricular vein, and in many cases ablation within the coronary sinus (CS) is necessary. Although RF ablation has proven to be feasible for the ablation of VTs and PVCs in the CS, the potential damage to the coronary arteries and the risk of cardiac tamponade make cryoablation an appealing alternative option. Obel *et al.*[16] reported on five patients successfully ablated in the CS with cryoenergy after the failure of RF.

However, in our study, cryoablation demonstrated limited effectiveness in targeting VAs arising from the CS. In fact, the stiffness of the cryocatheter hampered effective advancement through the distal CS in two of the cases, thus limiting its potential use. Cryoablation was also tested in the setting of structural heart disease.

Although in these patients a considerable amount of ablation is generally required (greater lesion depth and perforation are rare in infarct regions of dense fibrosis), cryoablation was considered due to the potentially higher risk of perforation in

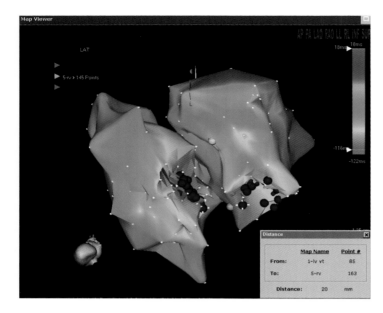

Figure 9.3. Electroanatomical (CARTO) map of a coronary cusp ventricular tachycardia (VT). Right ventricle and left ventricle in the left lateral view. The red dots indicate unsuccessful applications of RFCA with PR prolongation. The successful cryoablation site (not visible in the CARTO map) was at the level of the left coronary cusp.

structurally abnormal ventricles. However, our results showed that cryoablation was not as effective as intended.

One case report has shown the efficacy of cryoenegy in the pericardial space after the failure of RF on a scar-related VT case.[8]

Previously, Lusgarten et al. assessed the safety and efficacy of epicardial cryoablation in a closed-chest dog model[17] and showed that 4 min applications of cryoenergy at −90 °C achieved effective ventricular lesions without significant damage to the surrounding structures such as the coronary arteries. Epicardial fat is a major limitation to achieving adequate lesions by RF energy. Human fat tissue has different conductivity behavior to hot or cold thermal energy, so it is tempting to hypothesize that cryoenergy would result in deeper lesions than RF ablation in the presence of epicardial fat due to the different conductivity behavior of human fat tissue to hot or cold thermal energy.[18,19]

Conclusions

Overall, cryoenergy for ablation of VA has shown only moderate success. Cryoablation represents an alternative energy source to reduce complications during ablation of VTs originating from sites close to other relevant cardiac structures, such as the coronary sinus, phrenic nerve, AV node, and coronary artery. In rare cases, cryoenergy can also be considered epicardially when RFCA has failed. These considerations arose from nonrandomized studies and from data that should be considered as pilot guides for further investigations.

In addition, the available data fail to completely represent the real-world VT population because the majority of the patients were generally healthier than the patients undergoing VT ablation.

References

1. Soejima K, Suzuki M, Maisel WH, et al. Catheter ablation in patients with multiple and unstable ventricular tachycardias after myocardial infarction: short ablation lines guided by reentry circuit isthmuses and sinus rhythm mapping. Circulation. 2001;104: 664–9.
2. Marchlinski FE, Callans DJ, Gottlieb CD, et al. Linear ablation lesions for control of unmappable ventricular tachycardia in patients with ischemic and nonischemic cardiomyopathy. Circulation. 2000;101: 1288–96.
3. Stevenson WG, Wilber DJ, Natale A, et al. Irrigated radiofrequency catheter ablation guided by electro-anatomic mapping for recurrent ventricular tachycardia after myocardial infarction: the multicenter thermocool ventricular tachycardia ablation trial. Circulation. 2008;118:2773–82.

4. De Ponti R. Cryothermal energy ablation of cardiac arrhythmias 2005: state of the art. Indian Pacing Electrophysiol J. 2005;5:12–24.

5. Khairy P, Chauvet P, Lehmann J, et al. Lower incidence of thrombus formation with cryoenergy versus radiofrequency catheter ablation. Circulation. 2003;107:2045–50.

6. Di Biase L, Al-Ahmad A, Santangeli P, et al. Safety and outcomes of cryoablation for ventricular tachyarrhythmias: results from a multicenter experience. Heart Rhythm. 2011;8:968–74.

7. Timmermans C, Manusama R, Alzand B, et al. Catheter-based cryoablation of postinfarction and idiopathic ventricular tachycardia: initial experience in a selected population. J Cardiovasc Electrophysiol. 2010;21:255–61.

8. Di Biase L, Saliba WI, Natale A. Successful ablation of epicardial arrhythmias with cryoenergy after failed attempts with radiofrequency energy. Heart Rhythm. 2009;6:109–12.

9. Gage AA, Baust J. Mechanisms of tissue injury in cryosurgery. Cryobiology. 1998;37:171–86.

10. Lister JW, Hoffman BF, Kavaler F. Reversible cold block of the specialized cardiac tissues of the unanaesthetized dog. Science. 1964;145:723–5.

11. Harrison L, Gallagher JJ, Kasell J, et al. Cryosurgical ablation of the A-V node–His bundle: a new method for producing A-V block. Circulation. 1977;55:463–70.

12. Klein GJ, Guiraudon GM, Perkins DG, et al. Surgical correction of the Wolff–Parkinson–White syndrome in the closed heart using cryosurgery: a simplified approach. J Am Coll Cardiol. 1984;3:405–9.

13. Dubuc M, Khairy P, Rodriguez-Santiago A, et al. Catheter cryoablation of the atrioventricular node in patients with atrial fibrillation: a novel technology for ablation of cardiac arrhythmias. J Cardiovasc Electrophysiol. 2001;12:439–44.

14. Hass GM, Taylor CB. A quantitative hypothermal method for production of local injury to tissue. Fed Proc. 1947;6:393.

15. Skanes AC, Klein G, Krahn A, et al. Cryoablation: potentials and pitfalls. J Cardiovasc Electrophysiol. 2004;15:S28–S34.

16. Obel OA, d'Avila A, Neuzil P, et al. Ablation of left ventricular epicardial outflow tract tachycardia from the distal great cardiac vein. J Am Coll Cardiol. 2006;48:1813–7.

17. Lustgarten DL, Bell S, Hardin N, et al. Safety and efficacy of epicardial cryoablation in a canine model. Heart Rhythm. 2005;2:82–90.

18. Hatfield HS, Puch LG. Thermal conductivity of human fat and muscle. Nature. 1951;168:918–9.

19. Tarlochan F, Ramesh S. Heat transfer model for predicting survival time in cold water immersion. Biomed Eng Appl Basis Commun. 2005;17:159–66.

CHAPTER 10

Catheter Cryoablation for the Treatment of Miscellaneous Arrhythmias

Ngai-Yin Chan

Princess Margaret Hospital, Hong Kong, China

Cryothermic lesion, compared with radiofrequency (RF) lesion, is less likely to cause collateral damage.[1] Catheter ablation of uncommon arrhythmias like focal atrial tachycardia (FAT) and inappropriate sinus tachycardia (IST) may require the creation of lesions close to other cardiac structures, including the atrioventricular node (AVN), phrenic nerve, coronary sinus (CS), ostia of pulmonary veins (PVs), and superior vena cava (SVC). The biophysical properties of cryothermic lesion make it a potentially more favorable energy source in ablating these substrates. On the other hand, atrioventricular nodal ablation (AVNA) is a highly effective procedure for rate control in patients with atrial fibrillation (AF) refractory to drug treatment. RF is a well-established energy source to achieve AVNA. However, the electromagnetic interference (EMI) inherent to RF is a potential drawback for patients with a cardiac implantable electronic device (CIED).

In this chapter, the data on RF catheter ablation (RFCA) in treating FAT and IST will be reviewed with special emphasis on its limitations. Data on AVNA by RF will also be described. The use of an alternative source of energy, cryothermy, in the treatment of these miscellaneous arrhythmias will then be discussed in detail with regard to its poten-tial advantages, practical application, current data, and limitations.

Electrophysiological characteristics and anatomical locations of focal atrial tachycardia

Regular atrial tachycardia is currently classified into either focal or macro-reentry types.[2] FAT is defined as atrial activation originating from a discrete focus, arbitrarily taken as <2 cm in diameter, with centrifugal spread. It accounts for up to 10% of all supraventricular tachycardia.[3] Data on the use of pharmacological therapy in FAT are limited and in general showed poor response with potential risk of side effects.[4–12] Consequently, catheter abla-tion has evolved to be the mainstay treatment for FAT. The underlying electrophysiological mecha-nisms of FAT include abnormal automaticity, trig-gered activity, and micro-reentry. FAT often arises without the presence of structural heart disease and with normal histology.[13] However, it was also reported by McGuire et al. that in patients undergo-ing surgical treatment for atrial tachycardia, nearly half of the resected specimens showed some degree of myocyte hypertrophy, inflammatory infiltration, fibrosis, or fatty substitution.[14] The exact mechanism for a particular FAT is not of much significance to an ablationist since the ablation strategy is to target a lesion to the anatomical focus of the arrhythmia irrespective of the underlying electrophysiological mechanism.

The anatomical locations of FAT tend to cluster at characteristic sites. These sites are where there is marked anisotropic conduction or the presence of atrial myocytes with nodal-like electrophysiological properties. The crista terminalis is the commonest site for FAT and contributes around two-thirds of all right-sided FAT.[15] As for the left atrial foci, the commonest sites are at the ostia of PVs.[16] Medi *et al.* reported the frequency of anatomical locations of FAT in a large retrospective series of 345 patients.[17] They found the following frequencies: crista terminalis (30%), tricuspid valve annulus (19%), PV ostia (16%), perinodal region (14%), CS (10%), atrial appendage (7%), and mitral valve annulus (5%).

Efficacy and safety of radiofrequency catheter ablation of FAT

RFCA is in general an effective treatment for FAT with low complication and recurrence rates. Acute procedural success rates from 69% to 100% have been reported from different ablation series.[18–22] With the advent of three-dimensional (3D) mapping techniques, the acute procedural success rate has increased significantly.[23] Chen *et al.* analyzed 16 studies on FAT ablation and identified right atrial focus as the only independent predictor of procedural success.[24] Despite the overall success and safety of RFCA in treating FAT, there is a potential risk of collateral damage to important cardiac or noncardiac structures in catheter ablation at some locations. High procedural success with low complication and recurrence rates were reported in small series of patients undergoing RFCA for FAT at different sites.[15,16,25–34] However, in real-life clinical practice, a significant proportion of patients are regarded as not suitable for RFCA because of the anatomic location of arrhythmic focus. Medi *et al.* reported that in 3.5% of patients with FAT, RFCA was not attempted because of close proximity of the AVN.[17] On the other hand, collateral damage did occur during RFCA for FAT. Anguera *et al.* reported one patient with transient phrenic nerve palsy after

RFCA for right lateral FAT and one patient complicated with complete heart block necessitating pacemaker implantation after RFCA for low right septal FAT.[20] In a study on RFCA for drug-resistant FAT in 12 patients, one patient developed transient suppression of the sinus node (SN) function, which recovered within 72 h.[35] In another study with 45 patients undergoing RFCA for FAT, 2 patients with foci near the SN and at the mid-right atrium developed transient suppression of SN function with junctional escape rhythm after ablation.[36] These two patients required temporary pacing, and the SN function returned after 23 and 58 h, respectively. The recurrence rate varies from 0% to 33% according to different series.[18] According to an analysis from multiple studies by Chen *et al.*, the overall recurrence rate was 7% and the risk factors for recurrence included older age, the presence of structural heart disease, and multiple foci of atrial tachycardia.[24]

Catheter cryoablation treatment for "high-risk" FAT

FAT may occur at "high-risk" locations where collateral damage to other intracardiac or extracardiac structures would potentially complicate an ablation procedure. These high-risk locations include the perinodal region, cristal terminalis or superior vena caval area adjacent to the phrenic nerve, SN, PV ostia, CS, and noncoronary aortic cusp. Catheter cryoablation is an alternative approach to treat high-risk FAT by creating a more accurate lesion with less chance of collateral damage. Cryolesion is characterized by disruption of membranous organelles with preservation of the myocardial architecture[37] and intact endothelial layer with minimal thrombus formation.[38] The accuracy of placing an ablation lesion is enhanced by the properties of "cryomapping" and cryoadhesion. In addition, although the lesion size of cryoablation is governed by multiple factors, it is in general smaller than that created by RF.[39] The capability of producing a reversible electrophysiological effect at a catheter tip temperature of −30 °C is termed "cryomapping." If the reversible electrophysiological effect is regarded as desirable, a permanent lesion can be created by lowering the catheter tip temperature further to −75 °C.

Unfortunately, data on the use of catheter cryoablation in FAT are quite scarce.[40,41] Bastani *et al.*

described their experience of cryoablation in 26 patients with high-risk FAT.[42] Seven of these patients had previously failed RFCA. The foci of FAT were close to the AVN in 14 patients, in the vicinity of the SN in 7 patients, and at the crista terminalis adjacent to the phrenic nerve in 5 patients. A 6 mm tip cryocatheter was used with cryomapping before ablation, and cryoablation of 240 s in duration was delivered with successful cryomapping. They achieved an acute procedural success rate of 96% and a recurrence rate of 12%. They reported two patients with transient phrenic nerve palsy that subsided after 1 day and 5 months, respectively.

Although no PV stenosis was reported in a small study on RFCA for FAT at PV ostia,[16] it is a well-known complication when RF current is delivered to the ostia of PV during AF ablation procedures.[43,44] Tse et al. has shown that by using cryoablation to perform segmental isolation of PV in the treatment of AF, the complication of PV stenosis could be prevented.[45] It is conceivable that, likewise, cryothermy is a safer energy source for ablation of FAT originating from PV ostia.

RFCA for FAT arising from SVC may be complicated with SN dysfunction or phrenic nerve palsy.[46] Dib et al. tested the use of cryoablation in the SVC during AF ablation procedures.[47] In seven patients who required SVC ablation as part of the AF ablation procedures, the phrenic nerve was stimulated by pacing at 4 cm distal to the SVC–right atrial junction. "Cryomapping" was performed at the target ablation site before cryoablation with a 4 mm tip catheter. Successful cryoablation was performed in six patients. In one patient, diaphragmatic contraction was observed to be impaired during "cryomapping," and cryoablation was not performed. Phrenic nerve function recovered promptly after termination of "cryomapping." The same ablation strategy may be used for FAT arising from the SVC. Figure 10.1 demonstrates an example of SVC isolation by a cryoballoon in a patient with SVT AT and AF.

Badhwar et al.[34] and Kistler et al.[28] reported experience in RFCA for AT arising from the CS body and ostium in 8 and 13 patients, respectively. They could achieve a high acute procedural success rate and no recurrence rate. There was only one complication of pericarditis. However, from the experience of RFCA inside the CS for epicardial accessory pathways, complications of CS thrombosis and coronary artery damage have been observed in both animal and human studies.[48–50] However, RFCA inside the CS is commonly associated with significant pain.[48] In contrast, cryoablation inside the CS (Figure 10.2) has been shown to be free of the complication of coronary artery damage.[51]

FAT may uncommonly occur at the noncoronary aortic sinus (NCAC). Ouyang et al. performed RFCA at the NCAC in nine patients with FAT.[52] They achieved procedural success in all patients without any complication and recurrence. In an animal study comparing different energy sources for aortic cusp ablation, disruption of elastic fibers in the aortic media was seen only after standard and cooled-tip RFCA but not cryoablation.[53] The size of the lesions was comparable between the cryoablation (6 mm tip catheter) and standard RFCA (4 mm tip catheter) groups. Lesions created by cooled-tip RFCA (4 mm tip catheter) were significantly larger than those created by the other two energy sources. Cryothermy may be a safer energy source to use for ablation in the NCAC.

Radiofrequency and cryothermal ablation for inappropriate sinus tachycardia

IST is a clinical syndrome characterized by nonparoxysmal palpitations at rest or early during exercise disproportional to the physiological needs.[54–58] The manifestations of this clinical syndrome are variable and diverse, with young women mostly affected. The symptoms vary from intermittent palpitations to other nonspecific ones including lightheadedness, chest pain, headache, myalgia, dyspnea, fatigue, presyncope, syncope, orthostatic intolerance, abdominal discomfort, anxiety, and depression.[59] For diagnosis of this condition, the mean 24 h or daytime heart rate has to exceed 95 beats per minute or the sinus rate has to increase by >25–30 beats per minute with a change from supine to standing position. In addition, the P-wave morphology is nearly identical to that of sinus rhythm during tachycardia. Even with these seemingly quantitative diagnostic criteria, IST remains an elusive diagnosis.[60] The prevalence of this condition has been reported to be 1.1% in a middle-aged population.[61]

The underlying mechanism of IST is poorly understood. Various mechanisms have been proposed. These include autonomic imbalance with

(a)

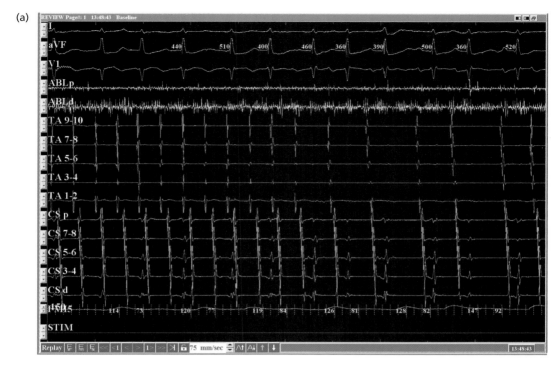

(b)

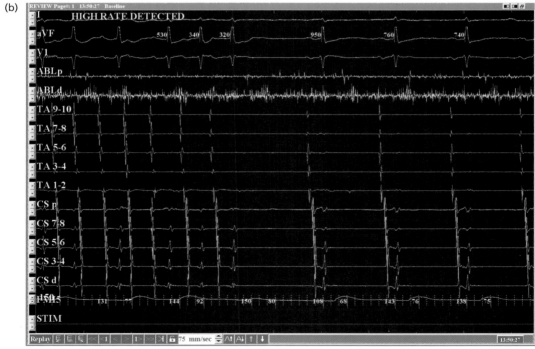

Figure 10.1. Electrical isolation of the superior vena cava (SVC) by a 28 mm cryoballoon in a patient with SVC atrial tachycardia (AT) and atrial fibrillation. (a) Slowing of SVC AT on initiation of cryoablation. (b) Termination of SVC AT during cryoablation. (c) Fluoroscopic position of the cryoballoon catheter in the right anterior oblique (RAO) view. The phrenic nerve was not captured with highest output at multiple areas. Diaphragmatic contraction was monitored by frequent fluoroscopic monitoring. (d) Fluorosopic position of the cryoballoon catheter in the left anterior oblique (LAO) view.

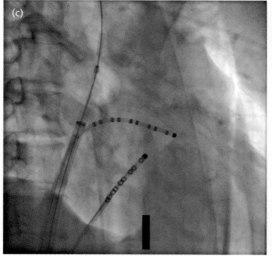
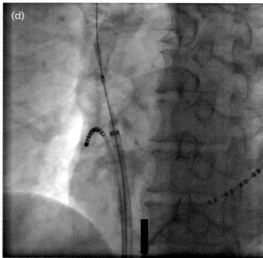

Figure 10.1. (*Continued*)

excessive sympathetic output or reduced parasym-pathetic influences, an excessive intrinsic sinus rate, ectopic activity of the SN, and the presence of β-receptor antibodies.[54,56,62] Treatment of IST is notoriously difficult.[60] The mainstay of treatment is pharmacological by the use of β-blockers. However, many patients are still symptomatic despite the use of maximal doses of β-blockers and other medications, including calcium channel blockers, clonidine, pyrodystigamine, and serotonin-reuptake inhibitors. Cappato *et al.* recently reported a randomized controlled study comparing ivabra-dine with placebo in the treatment of IST.[63] Ivabra-dine[64,65] is a specific blocker of I_f current, which is the ionic current known to generate the spontaneous diastolic depolarization of the sinoatrial node.[66] They found that patients taking ivabradine reported elimination of >70% of symptoms, and 47% of them experienced complete resolution of symptoms.

Sinus node modification by RFCA is an accepted treatment option for patients with drug-refractory IST. Different ablation techniques with the use of activation mapping, 3D nonfluoroscopic mapping, and noncontact mapping and with the help of Intracardiac echocardiography have been reported.[67-70] A combined endocardial and epicar-dial ablation strategy[71] and surgical approach[72] have also been described in case reports. Although high acute procedural success rates could be achieved with SN modification by RFCA, a significant propor-tion of patients had persistence of symptoms and

documented recurrence of IST. Marrouche *et al.* per-formed SN modification in 39 patients with IST with a 3D nonfluoroscopic mapping system; they achieved a 100% acute procedural success rate. However, 44% of the patients had persistence of symptoms, and 21% had documented recur-rence.[69] Furthermore, SN modification by RFCA is also associated with potential complications of SVC syndrome, phrenic nerve palsy, and SN dysfunction necessitating permanent pacemaker implantation.[69,70,73-75]

Catheter cryoablation is an alternative ablation strategy for the treatment of IST. As discussed in the "Catheter Cryoablation Treatment for 'High-Risk' FAT" section, cryothermy has less risk of causing collateral damage compared with RF and may be a better energy source in SN modification. Unfortu-nately, the data in this area are extremely scarce. Friedman *et al.* reported the successful use of an 8 mm tip cryocatheter in the modification of SN in a patient with IST.[76] A steerable 20-pole "halo" catheter was positioned in the right atrium with the proximal poles in the SVC–right atrial junction, the middle poles along the lateral right atrial wall, and the distal poles traversing the cavotricuspid isthmus and proximal CS. The site of earliest atrial activa-tion during isoproterenol infusion was targeted, and a 4 min cryoapplication was delivered. The patient remained symptom free after one year, and there was also objective evidence of subsidence of IST with Holter monitoring. Radu-Gabriel *et al.*

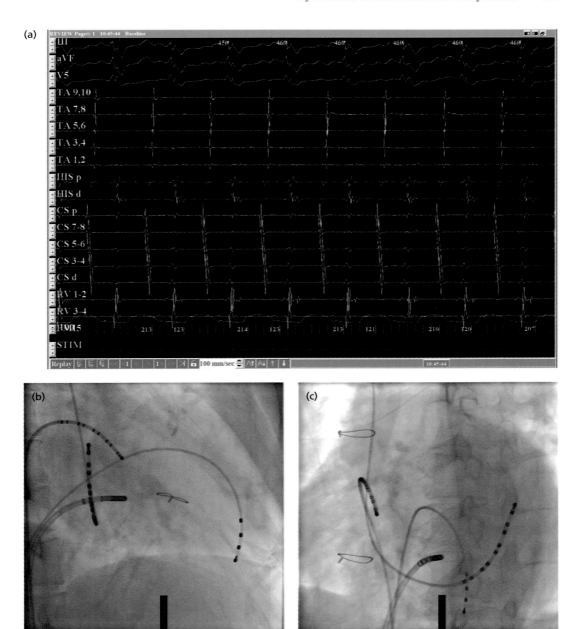

Figure 10.2. Catheter cryoablation in a patient with focal atrial tachycardia arising from the ostium of the coronary sinus. (a) Focal atrial tachycardia with earliest atrial activation at the ostium of the coronary sinus. (b) Fluoroscopic position of an 8 mm cryocatheter placed at the ostium of the coronary sinus during ablation in the right anterior oblique (RAO) view. (c) Fluoroscopic position of an 8 mm cryocatheter placed at the ostium of the coronary sinus during ablation in the left anterior oblique (LAO) view.

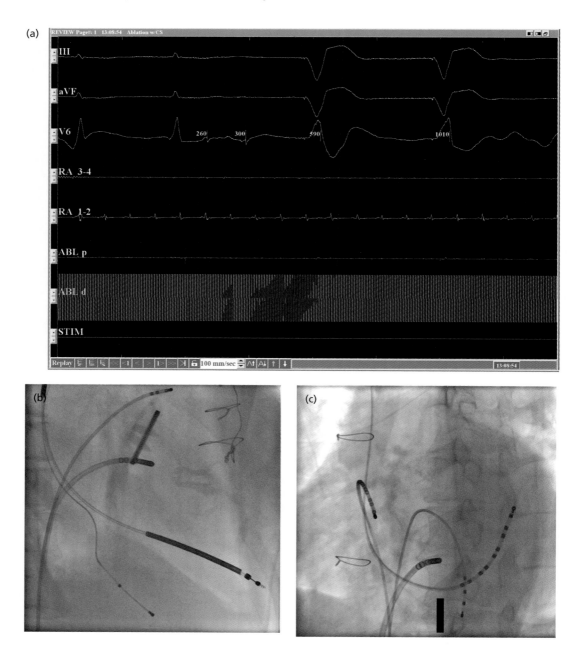

Figure 10.3. Atrioventricular nodal ablation (AVNA) by cryoablation using an 8 mm cryocatheter in a patient with atrial fibrillation and implantation of a cardiac resynchronization therapy defibrillator. (a) AVNA achieved during cryoablation. Note the characteristic artifacts arising from ice ball formation at the tip of the cryocatheter. (b) Fluoroscopic position of the 8 mm cryocatheter at the atrioventricular junction during ablation in the right anterior oblique (RAO) view. (c) Fluoroscopic position of the 8 mm cryocatheter at the atrioventricular junction during ablation in the left anterior oblique (LAO) view view.

reported another successful case of SN modification by cryoablation in a patient with IST.[77] However, the procedure was complicated by asymptomatic right phrenic nerve palsy, which only partially recovered at 2 months.

Radiofrequency and cryothermal ablation for atrioventricular nodal ablation in atrial fibrillation

Atrioventricular nodal ablation together with permanent pacemaker implantation is a recommended therapeutic option for rate control in patients with AF when pharmacological treatment fails to control the ventricular rate adequately.[78] (See Video Clip 10.1.) It has been shown by various studies that this strategy resulted in improvement of cardiac symptoms, quality of life, and health care utilization in patients with symptomatic AF refractory to drugs.[79–83] Radiofrequency is the predominant energy source used for AVNA in both studies and clinical practice. Although RF is a highly effective energy source for AVNA, the generation of EMI may be problematic in patients with CIEDs like pacemakers and implantable cardioverter defibrillators (ICDs). Previous studies have shown a high incidence (up to 53%) of pacemaker dysfunction caused by EMI during RFCA.[84] Despite reprogramming of the devices before ablation, permanent damage to leads and devices have been reported.[85] In that study, a progressive rise in the pacing threshold of ICD leads has been observed in 15% of patients undergoing AVNA by RF.

AVNA by cryothermy has the advantage of being free of EMI, and the potential risk in patients with CIEDs is thus avoided.[86] However, the reported experience in this area is limited. Friedman et al. performed AVNA with a 4 mm tip cryocatheter in 12 patients with AF. The acute procedural success rate was only 67%. In my experience, a high acute procedural success rate comparable to that of RF can be achieved with the use of an 8 mm tip cryocatheter (Figure 10.3).

Conclusions

Focal atrial tachycardia can occur at high-risk locations, and RFCA may cause collateral damage to cardiac or noncardiac structures. The procedures may also be aborted because of the anticipated

risks. Catheter cryoablation may be a more suitable treatment strategy for high-risk FAT, with potentially less risk for collateral damage. However, there are only limited data in this area. Similarly, SN modification by RFCA in the treatment of IST may be complicated by SVC syndrome, phrenic nerve palsy, and SN dysfunction. Catheter cryoablation may be considered in an attempt to avoid these complications. Lastly, in patients with CIEDs, EMI from RF delivered to perform AVNA or RFCA itself may transiently or permanently damage the device. Cryothermy may be a safer energy source in achieving AVNA in patients with CIEDs.

 Interactive Case Studies related to this chapter can be found at this book's companion website, at **www.chancryoablation.com**

References

1. Chan NY. The practice of catheter cryoablation for cardiac arrhythmias. Hoboken, NJ: Wiley Blackwell; 2013.
2. Saoudi N, Cosio F, Waldo A, et al. A classification of atrial flutter and regular atrial tachycardia according to electrophysiological mechanisms and anatomical bases; a statement from a Joint Expert Group from the Working Group of Arrhythmias of the European Society of Cardiology and the North American Society of Pacing and Electrophysiology. Eur Heart J. 2001;22:1162–82.
3. Porter MJ, Morton JB, Denman R, et al. Influence of age and gender on the mechanism of supraventricular tachycardia. Heart Rhythm. 2004;1:393–6.
4. Blomström-Lundqvist C, Scheinman MM, Aliot EM, et al. ACC/AHA/ESC guidelines for the management of patients with supraventricular arrhythmias. J Am Coll Cardiol. 2003;42:1493–531.
5. Mehta AV, Sanchez GR, Sacks EJ, et al. Ectopic automatic atrial tachycardia in children: clinical characteristics, management and follow-up. J Am Coll Cardiol. 1988;11:379–85.
6. Kunze KP, Kuck KH, Schluter M, et al. Effect of encainide and flecainide on chronic ectopic atrial tachycardia. J Am Coll Cardiol. 1986;7:1121–26.
7. Kuck KH, Kunze KP, Schluter M, et al. Encainide versus flecainide for chronic atrial and junctional ectopic tachycardia. Am J Cardiol. 1988;62: 37L–44L.
8. Pool PE, Quart BD. Treatment of ectopic atrial arrhythmias and premature atrial complexes in

adults with encainide. Am J Cardiol. 1988;62: 60L–62L.

9. Prager NA, Cox JL, Lindsay BD, *et al*. Long-term effectiveness of surgical treatment of ectopic atrial tachycardia. J Am Coll Cardiol. 1993;22:85–92.

10. Berns E, Rinkenberger RL, Jeang MK, *et al*. Efficacy and safety of flecainide acetate for atrial tachycardia and fibrillation. Am J Cardiol. 1987;59:1337–41.

11. Guccione P, Paul T, Garson A Jr. Long-term follow-up of amiodarone therapy in the young: continued efficacy, unimpaired growth, moderate side effects. J Am Coll Cardiol. 1990;15:1118–24.

12. Coumel P, Fidelle J. Amiodarone in the treatment of cardiac arrhythmias in children: one hundred thirty-five cases. Am Heart J. 1980;100(6 Pt. 2):1063–9.

13. Rosso R, Kistler PM. Focal atrial tachycardia. Heart. 2010;96:181–5.

14. McGuire MA, Johnson DC, Nunn GR, *et al*. Surgical therapy for atrial tachycardia in adults. J Am Coll Cardiol. 1989;14:1777–82.

15. Kalman JM, Olgin JE, Karch MR, *et al*. "Cristal tachycardias": origin of right atrial tachycardias from the cristal terminalis identified by intracardiac echocardiography. J Am Coll Cardiol. 1998;31:451–9.

16. Kistler PM, Sanders P, Fynn SP, *et al*. Electrophysiological and electrocardiographic characteristics of focal atrial tachycardia originating from the pulmonary veins: acute and long-term outcomes of radiofrequency ablation. Circulation. 2003;108:1968–75.

17. Medi C, Kalman JM, Haggani H, *et al*. Tachycardia-mediated cardiomyopathy secondary to focal atrial tachycardia: long-term outcome after catheter ablation. J Am Coll Cardiol. 2009;53:1791–7.

18. Roberts-Thomson KC, Kistler PM, *et al*. Focal atrial tachycardia II: management. Pacing Clin Electrophysiol. 2006;29:769–78.

19. Lesh MD, Van Hare GF, Epstein LM, *et al*. Radiofrequency catheter ablation of atrial arrhythmias. Results and mechanisms. Circulation. 1994;89: 1074–89.

20. Anguera I, Brugada J, Roba M, *et al*. Outcomes after radiofrequency catheter ablation of atrial tachycardia. Am J Cardiol. 2001;87:886–90.

21. Poty H, Saoudi N, Haissaguerre M, *et al*. Radiofrequency catheter ablation of atrial tachycardias. Am Heart J. 1996;131:481–9.

22. Kammeraad JA, Balaji S, Oliver RP, *et al*. Nonautomatic focal atrial tachycardia: characterization and ablation of a poorly understood arrhythmia in 38 patients. Pacing Clin Electrophysiol. 2003;26: 736–42.

23. Natale A, Breeding L, Tomassoni G, *et al*. Ablation of right and left ectopic atrial tachycardias using a three-dimensional nonfluoroscopic mapping system. Am J Cardiol. 1998;82:989–92.

24. Chen SA, Tai CT, Chiang CE, *et al*. Focal atrial tachycardia: reanalysis of the clinical and electrophysiologic characteristics and prediction of successful radiofrequency ablation. J Cardiovasc Electrophysiol. 1998;9:355–65.

25. Morton JB, Sanders P, Das A, *et al*. Focal atrial tachycardia arising from the tricuspid annulus: electrophysiolgic and electrocardiographic characteristics. J Cardiovasc Electrophysiol. 2001;12:653–9.

26. Hachiya H, Ernst S, Ouyang F, *et al*. Topographic distribution of focal left atrial tachycardia defined by electrocardiographic and electrophysiological data. Circ J. 2005;69:205–10.

27. Kistler PM, Sanders P, Hussin A, *et al*. Focal atrial tachycardia arising from the mitral annulus: Electrocardiographic and electrophysiologic characterization. J Am Coll Cardiol. 2003;41:2212–19.

28. Kistler PM, Fynn SP, Haqqani H, *et al*. Focal atrial tachycardia from the ostium of the coronary sinus: electrocardiographic and electrophysiological characterization and radiofrequency ablation. J Am Coll Cardiol. 2005;45:1488–93.

29. Roberts-Thomson KC, Kistler PM, Haqqani HM, *et al*. Focal atrial tachycardias arising from the right atrial appendage: electrocardiographic and electrophysiologic characteristics and radiofrequency ablation. J Cardiovasc Electrophysiol. 2007;18:367–72.

30. Dong J, Schreieck J, Ndrepepa G, *et al*. Ectopic tachycardia originating from the superior vena cava. J Cardiovasc Electrophysiol. 2002;13:620–4.

31. Chen CC, Tai CT, Chiang CE, *et al*. Atrial tachycardias originating from the atrial septum: electrophysiologic characteristics and radiofrequency ablation. J Cardiovasc Electrophysiol. 2000;11:744–9.

32. Iesaka Y, Takahashi A, Goya M, *et al*. Adenosine-sensitive atrial re-entrant tachycardia originating from the atrioventricular nodal transitional area. J Cardiovasc Electrophysiol. 1997;8:854–64.

33. Lai LP, Lin JL, Chen TF, *et al*. Clinical, electrophysiological characteristics and radiofrequency catheter ablation of atrial tachycardia near the apex of Koch's triangle. Pacing Clin Electrophysiol. 1998;21: 367–74.

34. Badhwar N, Kalman JM, Sparks PB, *et al*. Atrial tachycardia arising from the coronary sinus musculature: electrophysiological characteristics and long-term outcomes of radiofrequency ablation. J Am Coll Cardiol. 2005;46:1921–30.

35. Walsh EP, Saul JP, Hulse JE, *et al*. Transcatheter ablation of ectopic atrial tachycardia in young patients using radiofrequency current. Circulation. 1992;86: 1138–46.

36. Pappone C, Stabile G, De Simone A, *et al*. Role of catheter-induced mechanical trauma in localization of target sites of radiofrequency ablation in auto-

matic atrial tachycardia. J Am Coll Cardiol. 1996;27: 1090–7.

37. Khairy P, Dubuc M. Transcatheter cryoablation part I: preclinical experience. Pacing Clin Electrophysiol. 2008;31:112–20.

38. Khairy P, Chauvet P, Lehmann J, et al. Lower incidence of thrombus formation with cryoenergy versus radiofrequency catheter ablation. Circulation. 2003; 107:2045–50.

39. Rodriguez LM, Leunissen J, Hoekstra A, et al. Transvenous cold mapping and cryoablation of the AV node in dogs: observations of chronic lesions and comparison to those obtained with radiofrequency ablation. J Cardiovasc Electrophysiol. 1998;9: 1055–61.

40. Wong T, Segal OR, Markides V, et al. Cryoablation of focal atrial tachycardia originating close to the atrioventricular node. J Cardiovasc Electrophysiol. 2004; 15:838.

41. Rodriguez LM, Geller JC, Tse HF, et al. Acute results of transvenous cryoablation of supraventricular tachycardia (atrial fibrillation, atrial flutter, Wolff–Parkinson–White syndrome, atrioventricular nodal re-entrant tachycardia). J Cardiovasc Electrophysiol. 2002;13:1082–9.

42. Bastani H, Insulander P, Schwieler J, et al. Safety and efficacy of cryoablation of atrial tachycardia with high risk of ablation-related injuries. Europace. 2009;11:625–9.

43. Yu WC, Hsu TL, Tai CT, et al. Acquired pulmonary vein stenosis after radiofrequency catheter ablation of paroxysmal atrial fibrillation. J Cardiovasc Electrophysiol. 2001;12:887–92.

44. Chen SA, Yu WC, Tai CT. Editorial comment: can we avoid pulmonary vein stenosis following ablation of atrial fibrillation? J Interv Card Electrophysiol. 2000;4:633–4.

45. Tse HF, Reek S, Timmermans C, et al. Pulmonary vein isolation using transvenous catheter cryoablation for treatment of atrial fibrillation without risk of pulmonary vein stenosis. J Am Coll Cardiol. 2003;42: 752–8.

46. Zhao ZH, Li XB, Guo J. Electrophysiologic characteristics of atrial tachycardia originating from the superior vena cava. J Interv Card Electrophysiol. 2009; 24:89–94.

47. Dib C, Kapa S, Powell BD, et al. Successful use of "cryomapping" to avoid phrenic nerve damage during ostial superior venal caval ablation despite nerve proximity. J Interv Card Electrophysiol. 2008;22: 23–30.

48. Haissagurre M, Gaita F, Fischer B, et al. Radiofrequency catheter ablation of left lateral accessory pathways via the coronary sinus. Circulation. 1992; 86:1464–8.

49. Langbery J, Griffin JC, Herre JM, et al. Catheter ablation of accessory pathways using radiofrequency energy in the canine coronary sinus. J Am Coll Cardiol. 1989;13:491–6.

50. Huang SK, Graham AR, Bharati S, et al. Short and long-term effects of transcatheter ablation of the coronary sinus by radiofrequency energy. Circulation. 1988;78:416–27.

51. Collins KK, Rhee EK, Kirsh JA, et al. Cryoablation of accessory pathways in the coronary sinus in young patients: a multicenter study from the Pediatric and Congenital Electrophysiology Society's Working Group on cryoablation. J Cardiovasc Electrophysiol. 2007;18:592–7.

52. Ouyang F, Ma J, Ho SY, et al. Focal atrial tachycardia originating from the non-coronary aortic sinus. J Am Coll Cardiol. 2006;48:122–31.

53. d'Avila A, Thiagalingam A, Holmvang G, et al. What is the most appropriate energy source for aortic cusp ablation? A comparison of standard RF, cooled-tip RF and cryothermal ablation. J Interv Card Electrophysiol. 2006;16:31–8.

54. Bauernfeind RA, Amat-Y-Leon F, Dhingra RC, et al. Chronic nonparoxysmal sinus tachycardia in otherwise healthy persons. Ann Intern Med. 1979;91: 702–10.

55. Krahn AD, Yee R, Klein GJ, et al. Inappropriate sinus tachycardia: evaluation and therapy. J Cardiovasc Electrophysiol. 1995;6:1124–8.

56. Morillo CA, Klein GJ, Thakur RK, et al. Mechanisms of inappropriate sinus tachycardia: role of sympathovagal imbalance. Circulation. 1994;90: 873–7.

57. Zipes D, Jalife J. Cardiac electrophysiology: from cell to bedside. 4th ed. Philadelphia, PA: Saunders; 2004.

58. Spodick DH, Raju P, Bishop RL, et al. Operational definition of normal sinus heart rate. Am J Cardiol. 1992;69:1245–6.

59. Shen WK, Low PA, Jahangir A, et al. Is sinus node modification appropriate for inappropriate sinus tachycardia with features of postural orthostatic tachycardia syndrome? Pacing Clin Electrophysiol. 2001; 24:217–30.

60. Shen WK. How to manage patients with inappropriate sinus tachycardia. Heart Rhythm. 2005;2: 1015–19.

61. Still AM, Raatikainen P, Ylitalo A, et al. Prevalence, characteristics and natural course of inappropriate sinus tachycardia. Europace. 2005;7:104–12.

62. Chiale PA, Garro HA, Schmidberg J, et al. Inappropriate sinus tachycardia may be related to an immunologic disorder involving adrenergic receptors. Heart Rhythm. 2006;3:1182–6.

63. Cappato R, Castelvecchio S, Ricci C, et al. Clinical efficacy of ivabradine in patients with inappropriate

sinus tachycardia. J Am Coll Cardiol. 2012;60: 1323–9.

64. Camm AJ, Lau CP. Electrophysiological effects of a single intravenous administration of ivabradine (S16257) in adult patients with normal baseline electrophysiology. Drugs R D. 2003;4:83–9.

65. Manz M, Reuter M, Lauck G, et al. A single intravenous dose of ivabradine, a novel I(f) inhibitor, lowers heart rate but does not depress left ventricular function in patients with left ventricular dysfunction. Cardiology. 2003;100:149–55.

66. DiFrancesco D. Pacemaker mechanisms in cardiac tissue. Annu Rev Physiol. 1993;55:455–72.

67. Lee RJ, Kalman JM, Fitzpatrick AP, et al. Radiofrequency catheter modification of the sinus node for "inappropriate" sinus tachycardia. Circulation. 1995;92:2919–28.

68. Man KC, Knight B, Tse HF, et al. Radiofrequency catheter ablation of inappropriate sinus tachycardia guided by activation mapping. J Am Coll Cardiol. 2000;35:451–7.

69. Marrouche NF, Beheiry S, Tomassoni G, et al. Three-dimensional nonfluoroscopic mapping and ablation of inappropriate sinus tachycardia: procedural strategies and long-term outcome. J Am Coll Cardiol. 2002; 39:1046–54.

70. Lin D, Garcia F, Jacobson J, et al. Use of noncontact mapping and saline-cooled ablation catheter for sinus node modification in medically refractory inappropriate sinus tachycardia. Pacing Clin Electrophysiol. 2007;30:236–42.

71. Koplan BA, Parkash R, Couper G, et al. Combined epicardial-endocardial approach to ablation of inappropriate sinus tachycardia. J Cardiovasc Electrophysiol. 2004;15:237–40.

72. Yee R, Guiraudon GM, Gardner MJ, et al. Refractory paroxysmal sinus tachycardia: management by subtotal right atrial exclusion. J Am Coll Cardiol. 1984;3:400–4.

73. Callans DJ, Ren JF, Schwartzman D, et al. Narrowing of the superior vena cava-right atrium junction during radiofrequency catheter ablation for inappropriate sinus tachycardia: analysis with intracardiac echocardiography. J Am Coll Cardiol. 1999;33: 1667–70.

74. Leonelli FM, Pisano E, Requarth JA, et al. Frequency of superior vena cava syndrome following radiofrequency modification of the sinus node and its management [brief report]. Am J Cardiol. 2000;85:771–4.

75. Durante-Mangoni E, Del Vecchio D, Ruggiero G. Right diaphragmatic paralysis following cardiac radiofrequency catheter ablation for inappropriate sinus tachycardia. Pacing Clin Electrophysiol. 2003;26:783–4.

76. Friedman PL, Bronson J, Macveigh TJ, et al. Sinus node modification using cryoenergy. Heart Rhythm. 2006;3:S255–6.

77. Vatasescu RGM, Shalganov TN, Jalabadze K, et al. Right diaphragmatic paralysis following endocardial cryothermal ablation of inappropriate sinus tachycardia. Heart Rhythm. 2006;3:S255.

78. Fuster V, Ryden LE, Cannom DS, et al. 2011 ACCF/AHA/HRS focused update incorporated into the ACC/AHA/ESC 2006 guidelines for the management of patients with atrial fibrillation. J Am Coll Cardiol. 2011;57:e101–98.

79. Brignole M, Menozzi C, Gianfranchi L, et al. Assessment of atrioventricular junction ablation and VVIR pacemaker versus pharmacological treatment in patients with heart failure and chronic atrial fibrillation: a randomized, controlled study. Circulation. 1998;98:953–60.

80. Brignole M, Gianfranchi L, Menozzi C, et al. Assessment of atrioventricular junction ablation and DDDR mode-switching pacemaker versus pharmacological treatment in patients with severely symptomatic paroxysmal atrial fibrillation: a randomized controlled study. Circulation. 1997;96:2617–24.

81. Kay GN, Ellenbogen KA, Giudici M, et al. The Ablate and Pace Trial: a prospective study of catheter ablation of the AV conduction system and permanent pacemaker implantation for treatment of atrial fibrillation. APT Investigators. J Interv Card Electrophysiol. 1998;2:121–35.

82. Wood MA, Brown-Mahoney C, Kay GN, et al. Clinical outcomes after ablation and pacing therapy for atrial fibrillation: a meta-analysis. Circulation. 2000;101: 1138–44.

83. Ozcan C, Jahangir A, Friedman PA, et al. Long-term survival after ablation of the atrioventricular node and implantation of a permanent pacemaker in patients with atrial fibrillation. N Engl J Med. 2001;344:1043–51.

84. Sadoul N, Blankoff I, de Chillou C, et al. Effects of radiofrequency catheter ablation on patients with permanent pacemakers. J Interv Card Electrophysiol. 1997;1:227–33.

85. Burke MC, Kopp DE, Alberts M, et al. Effect of radiofrequency current on previously implanted pacemaker and defibrillator ventricular lead systems. J Electrocardiol. 2001;34(Suppl.):143–8.

86. Siu CW, Tse HF, Lau CP. Avoidance of electromagnetic interference to implantable cardioverter-defibrillator during atrioventricular node ablation for atrial fibrillation using transvenous cryoablation. Pacing Clin Electrophysiol. 2006;29:914–16.

Index

Page numbers in *italics* denote figures, those in **bold** denote tables.

The Practice of Catheter Cryoablation for Cardiac Arrhythmias, First Edition. Edited by Ngai-Yin Chan.
© 2014 John Wiley & Sons, Ltd. Published 2014 by John Wiley & Sons, Ltd.